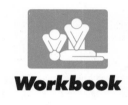

Workbook

American Red Cross CPR: Basic Life Support for the Professional Rescuer

ISBN: 0-86536-082-0

Acknowledgments

This course is based on the Standards and Guidelines established by the 1985 National Conference on Cardiopulmonary Resuscitation and Emergency Cardiac Care.

The course and this workbook are products of the 1987–1988 CPR/First Aid Project at Red Cross national headquarters. Members of the Basic Life Support development team included: Franklyn R. Greenberg, Ed.D., writer/designer; Mary F. Cotton, Ph.D., Jean E. Curran, Heddy F. Reid, Lawrence Newell, Ed.D., and Richard C. Havel, Ed.D. Additional assistance was provided by Program Development Division staff including: Bruce Spitz, director; Frank Carroll, Jessica Bernstein, M.P.H., Vikki Scott, M.P.A., and Susan Walter. The following national sector staff also provided review and assistance: Joan Handler, Alfred J. Katz, M.D., Carole Kauffman, R.N., John M. Malatak, M.S., and Thomas C. Werts.

Technical advice and review were provided by:
Warren D. Bowman, M.D., F.A.C.P., National Medical Adviser to the National Ski Patrol; Chairman, Medical Committee of the National Association for Search and Rescue.

Allan Braslow, Ph.D., Faculty, 1985 National Conference on CPR and Emergency Cardiac Care; Braslow & Associates.

John Clair, Assistant National Chairman, National Ski Patrol.

Douglas D'Arnall, U.S. Lifesaving Association Representative to the Council for National Cooperation in Aquatics; Beach Services Manager, Huntington Beach, Calif.

George E. Membrino, Ph.D., Associate Dean for Continuing Education and Associate Professor, Department of Family and Community Medicine, University of Massachusetts Medical School.

George Paraskos, M.D., Chairman, AHA–ECC Subcommittee; Associate Chairman and Professor of Medicine, University of Massachusetts Medical School.

William J. Schneiderman, Adjunct Clinical Instructor, Emergency Care Institute, NYU/Bellevue Hospital Center, and former Education Coordinator, Department of Emergency Medical Services, New York Infirmary–Beekman Downtown Hospital.

This manuscript also was reviewed by the National Academy of Sciences–National Research Council Committee to Advise the American National Red Cross.

Field representatives providing advice and guidance through the 1987–1988 Red Cross CPR Advisory Committee included:
W. Larry Bair, Central Iowa Chapter, Des Moines, Iowa
D. Earl Harbert, Field Service Manager, Wichita, Kan.
Jerry Hummel, Southeastern Michigan Chapter, Detroit, Mich.
Lonnie Kirby, Western Operations Headquarters, Burlingame, Calif.
Wanda Leffler, Indianapolis Area Chapter, Indianapolis, Ind.
Mary M. ("Posie") Mansfield, Danvers, Mass., Chair, Basic Life Support Sub-Committee of the CPR Advisory Committee
C. Ray McLain, R.N., M.S.N., University of Alabama at Birmingham, Birmingham, Ala.
Marshall Meyer, Oregon Trail Chapter, Portland, Oreg.
Gary J. Taylor, Greater Kansas City Chapter, Kansas City, Mo.
Richard Tulis, American Red Cross of Massachusetts Bay, Boston, Mass.
John Wagner, Albany Area Chapter, Albany, N.Y.

Red Cross chapters that participated in field tests included:
Albany Area Chapter, Albany, N.Y.
American Red Cross of Massachusetts Bay, Boston, Mass.
Central Iowa Chapter, Des Moines, Iowa
Greater Kansas City Chapter, Kansas City, Mo.
Greater New Bedford Chapter, New Bedford, Mass.
Mile High Chapter, Denver, Colo.
Santa Clara Valley Chapter, San Jose, Calif.
Southeastern Michigan Chapter, Detroit, Mich.

Groups participating in field tests included:
City of New Bedford Emergency Medical Services, New Bedford, Mass.
Des Moines Fire Recruits Class, Des Moines, Iowa
Detroit Edison Company, Detroit, Mich.
Environmental Safety Department, Hewlett Packard, San Jose, Calif.
Jewish Community Center, Albany, N.Y.
Lyons Ambulance Service Personnel, Danvers, Mass.
Nurses of the Community Blood Center of Greater Kansas City, Kansas City, Mo.

Preface

Since 1909, the American Red Cross has trained millions of Americans in first aid skills. In 1973, the Red Cross began teaching CPR skills to the lay public. Starting in 1986, the Red Cross began a major effort to revise all of its first aid and CPR courses and supporting materials to reflect up-to-date emergency care standards and new teaching approaches.

This new course is designed to meet the special needs of people who are expected to respond in emergency situations. It represents a new direction in CPR training set by the 1985 National Conference on Standards and Guidelines for Cardiopulmonary Resuscitation and Emergency Cardiac Care. This direction distinguishes the training needs of the lay public in fundamental CPR skills from the more advanced training needs of the group the American Red Cross now calls "professional rescuers."

This course presents advanced skills and information, presuming that course participants have already successfully completed fundamental CPR skills training. Satisfactory completion of this course results in American Red Cross certification in Basic Life Support for the Professional Rescuer.

This course will teach:

1. The role of the professional rescuer in providing emergency care and saving lives.
2. How to recognize and respond to cardiac and respiratory emergencies.
3. The risk factors that contribute to cardiovascular disease.
4. Specialized skills and techniques for two-rescuer CPR and special rescue situations, including the use of resuscitation masks.

The goal of the American Red Cross is to help people avoid, prepare for, and cope with emergencies. This course is offered to meet the needs and interests of those people the public expects to respond in an emergency.

The American Red Cross wishes to express its gratitude to the American Medical Association and the editors of *The Journal of the American Medical Association* for permission to reprint material and language from the "Standards and Guidelines for Cardiopulmonary Resuscitation and Emergency Cardiac Care," *The Journal of the American Medical Association,* 1986, Vol. 255, No. 21. Much of this course was developed around the recommendations set forth in those Standards and Guidelines.

The 1985 National Conference on Standards and Guidelines for Cardiopulmonary Resuscitation and Emergency Cardiac Care was sponsored by the American College of Cardiology, the American Heart Association, the American Red Cross, and the National Heart, Lung, and Blood Institute.

Contents

Workbook

This workbook includes several features to help participants learn new skills and material. They include:

Main Ideas Page

Each chapter begins with a page that lists the main ideas, followed by a chapter outline and a list of objectives. The main ideas introduce the major concepts on which the chapter outline is based. The objectives provide the participant with the skills or knowledge to be mastered.

Review

A review section is included at the end of each chapter. Answering the review questions will help participants learn the material, and help prepare them for the final test. Answers should be written in the workbook. The correct answers to each set of questions can be found on the page following the questions.

Skill Sheets

Some chapters include skill sheets that describe in detail how to perform certain CPR skills taught in this course. The skill sheets are used during practice sessions. Participants will practice with a partner and on a manikin.

Skill Checklists

Skill checklists are included for all CPR skills that require testing or checking out by the instructor. These checklists present a shortened version of the steps that are included in the detailed skill sheets. Each checklist includes the **critical skills** that participants must perform correctly in order to pass the skill tests.

Glossary

A glossary has been included at the end of the workbook to explain terms that may not be familiar. Words that are printed in bold type in the text are defined in the glossary.

Video/Films

During the course, participants will watch a series of short videos or films presenting medical emergencies and demonstrating the skills to be practiced. Watching the demonstrations closely will help participants perform the skills during the practice sessions.

Tests

There are two types of tests in this course: skill tests and written tests. Skill tests are given after participants have practiced a skill and are ready to be checked by the instructor. A written multiple choice test is given at the end of the course.

Part I: The Foundation for Professional Rescuer Skills

This course is divided into two parts. Part I, "The Foundation for Professional Rescuer Skills" (Chapters 1–5), addresses the role of the professional rescuer in providing basic life support (BLS) in an emergency. Part I also considers the importance of community *awareness* and *prevention* in reducing deaths from cardiovascular disease. Also discussed is the role of the professional rescuer as part of a community's emergency medical services (EMS) system.

The chapter on the respiratory and circulatory systems links the professional rescuer's knowledge of anatomy with the timely performance of such critical lifesaving skills as rescue breathing and CPR. A chapter about the risk factors associated with cardiovascular disease can help the professional rescuer examine his or her own lifestyle and diet, to encourage making the changes necessary to increase the chance of living longer. This chapter also discusses the signals of angina pectoris, heart attack, cardiac arrest, and stroke, as well as actions to take for these conditions.

During Part I, course participants are given a skill test where their knowledge of fundamental CPR skills is checked by the instructor. These skills include one-rescuer adult, child, and infant CPR, and first aid for airway obstruction in the conscious and unconscious adult and infant. Participants must demonstrate competency in these skills before they progress to Part II of the course.

Part II, "The Professional Rescuer Skills" (Disease Transmission Information and Chapters 6–9), presents a series of new skills for professional rescuers that build upon the foundation of single-rescuer skills. These include two-rescuer CPR, more advanced techniques for airway management, techniques for positioning and ventilating the victim of a suspected head, neck, or back injury, and use of a resuscitation mask. These skills are described in the workbook, shown in the films or videos, and taught through hands-on practice sessions.

Special guidelines for the professional rescuer on preventing disease transmission have been provided at the beginning of Part II. At the end of Part II is a chapter on how to respond to patients and give care in special resuscitation situations.

The appendix contains information on medicolegal considerations for professional rescuers. In addition, a glossary is provided to define terms that may be unfamiliar.

1

1 Basic Life Support and the Professional Rescuer

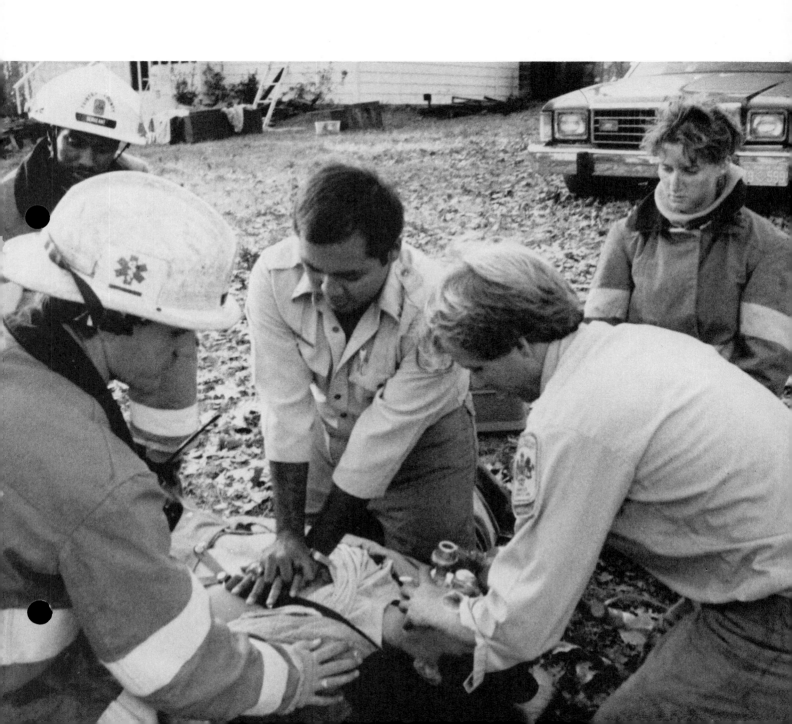

MAIN IDEAS

1. Professional rescuers serve their communities in many ways. They are trained to provide assistance in an emergency.
2. Cardiovascular disease is the leading cause of death in the United States.
3. Sudden death from heart attack is the most common fatal medical emergency today.
4. CPR *does* make a difference in saving lives.
5. Patient survival depends upon how quickly basic life support (BLS) and advanced cardiac life support (ACLS) are started.
6. This course prepares the professional rescuer to provide BLS in a respiratory or cardiac emergency.

CHAPTER OUTLINE

I. The Professional Rescuer
II. Cardiovascular Disease: The Nation's Leading Cause of Death
III. CPR Saves Lives
  A. The first critical moments
  B. The impact of CPR
IV. The Role of the Professional Rescuer and Basic Life Support
V. Review

OBJECTIVES

1. Identify and describe the leading cause of death in the United States.
2. Identify the critical times that increase the chances for saving a patient whose heart has stopped.
3. Describe what is expected of a professional rescuer at the scene of a medical emergency.

The Professional Rescuer

This course is designed for those individuals who have been, or are being, trained to assume responsibilities for delivering health care and/or assuring public safety. The roles of individuals who work as **professional rescuers** are varied and include the following:

- Allied health professionals (e.g., medical assistants, physical therapists, respiratory therapists, and X-ray technicians)
- Athletic trainers
- Business and industry safety personnel
- Emergency medical technicians (EMTs)
- Firefighters
- Flight attendants
- Lifeguards
- Members of search and rescue teams
- Nurses
- Paramedics
- Park rangers
- Physicians
- Police officers
- Public safety personnel
- Security personnel
- Ski patrollers

Professional rescuers are people who serve their communities as volunteers, as well as those who are paid for their work. Although professional rescuers have many different occupations, they share two important characteristics:
- They have a duty when they are on the job to respond in an emergency.
- They have been professionally trained and use certain techniques that are not generally taught in CPR courses offered to the general public.

Cardiovascular Disease: The Nation's Leading Cause of Death

Cardiovascular disease affects a large portion of the population and is associated with heart attack, stroke, and high blood pressure. Every year, nearly one million people die from some form of cardiovascular disease *(Fig. 1)*—over one-half of them from **coronary heart disease.** This form of cardiovascular disease is the cause of heart attack, the most common medical emergency leading to sudden death.

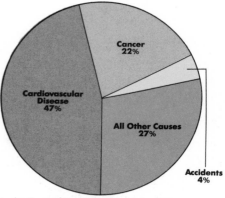

Leading Causes of Death in the United States—1985
Total Number of Deaths = 2,086,440

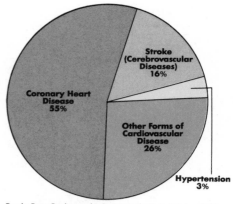

Deaths From Cardiovascular Disease in the United States—1985
Total Number of Deaths From Cardiovascular Disease = 977,879

Figure 1
The Leading Causes of Death in the United States—1985
Deaths From Cardiovascular Disease in the United States—1985[1]

Almost everyone has been touched in some way by the impact of cardiovascular disease. Most people enrolled in this course probably know someone who has been a victim of some form of this disease. Some people sitting in this room already have this disease. The seriousness of the problem is illustrated by the following facts.

Facts About Cardiovascular Disease

- One out of every two deaths in the United States is due to cardiovascular disease.
- Cardiovascular disease accounts for almost one million deaths annually in the United States.
- Coronary heart disease claims approximately 500,000 lives every year, with the majority of these being sudden deaths.
- Two-thirds of sudden deaths due to coronary heart disease take place outside of a hospital. These deaths most often occur within two hours after the onset of symptoms.

CPR Saves Lives

Since its introduction in 1960 as a lifesaving skill, cardio-pulmonary resuscitation (CPR) has made a significant difference in reducing premature deaths from cardiovascular disease. CPR is an emergency procedure used for a person who is not breathing and whose heart has stopped beating.

CPR is one of the components of **basic life support (BLS).** For the purposes of this course, BLS includes rescue breathing, obstructed airway management, CPR, and, when appropriate, activating the emergency medical services (EMS) system.

Time is a critical factor in saving the lives of victims of cardiac arrest. When a patient's heart has stopped, his or her survival depends on how quickly CPR is started and how quickly the patient receives **advanced cardiac life support (ACLS).** ACLS includes BLS plus advanced airway management, interpretation of heart rhythms displayed on a cardiac monitor, **defibrillation,** establishment of an intravenous line, and the administration of cardiac drugs.

Medical authorities indicate that the greatest number of lives can be saved in cardiac emergencies if BLS is started within 3 to 4 minutes after the heart stops. CPR must then be followed by ACLS within 10 minutes after the heart stops[2] *(Fig. 2).*

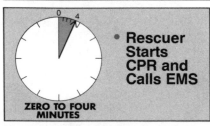

- **Victim's Heart Stops**

ZERO MINUTES

- **Rescuer Starts CPR and Calls EMS**

ZERO TO FOUR MINUTES

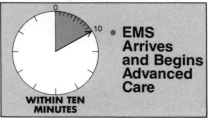

- **EMS Arrives and Begins Advanced Care**

WITHIN TEN MINUTES

Figure 2
Critical Times for Saving a Life

The effectiveness of CPR in saving lives has been well documented. As noted at the 1985 National Conference on Standards and Guidelines for Cardiopulmonary Resuscitation and Emergency Cardiac Care—

- Persons who receive CPR right after the heart stops have the best chance of survival.
- If CPR is rapidly followed by ACLS, some 40 percent of the patients can be saved.
- In certain studies, CPR followed by ACLS was successful in more than 60 percent of cases in bringing about successful resuscitation.

The Professional Rescuer and Basic Life Support

The professional rescuer is frequently the first trained person to respond to a medical emergency. He or she plays an important role in the emergency care of the patient, whether the emergency happens in the community (pre-hospital) or in the hospital. The professional rescuer helps save lives, prevents additional injuries, and comforts the patient(s) until more advanced medical assistance arrives.

Basic life support is the first level of care needed to keep a patient alive in a life-threatening emergency and includes those skills necessary to maintain breathing and circulation. This course includes BLS techniques that enable the rescuer to recognize and assist a victim of the following emergencies:

Respiratory Emergency
In a respiratory emergency, a person is having difficulty breathing, or is in **respiratory arrest.**

Cardiac Emergency
In a cardiac emergency, a person's heart is not functioning properly. Two common cardiac emergencies are heart attack and cardiac arrest.

Another common type of cardiac emergency that the professional rescuer needs to know about is **angina pectoris.** This condition is discussed in Chapter 4.

Professional rescuers are a vital part of the EMS system, a community network providing immediate assistance to a victim in a medical emergency. In many cases, the professional rescuer is dispatched to the scene of an emergency as part of the EMS system. Another responsibility of the professional rescuer providing BLS is to contact the EMS system if the emergency occurs in a pre-hospital setting, and if he or she has not been dispatched to the scene as part of the EMS system. For example, a lifeguard who rescues someone who is drowning, or a police officer who discovers a car accident, must activate the EMS system.

When the professional rescuer arrives at the scene of an emergency, he or she must first survey the scene to determine if there is any danger to the patient, the rescuer, or bystanders. After determining that the scene is safe, the rescuer immediately assesses the patient's condition. The most important priorities in this initial patient assessment are checking to see that *the patient has an open airway, is breathing, that the heart is beating, and that there is no severe bleeding. Note:* "Severe bleeding" is arterial bleeding—bleeding that spurts from a wound with every beat of the heart—and is the only bleeding that needs to be controlled *immediately.* The rescuer should first check for a pulse, then control any severe bleeding.

Where necessary, the professional rescuer may play a key role in seeing that advanced cardiac life support (ACLS) reaches the patient as soon as possible. He or she calls the EMS dispatcher and reports or confirms the patient's condition and circumstances of the emergency.

Professional rescuers have a critical part to play in providing emergency care to the victim of a respiratory or cardiac emergency. The prompt response of professional rescuers is one part of a community approach to reducing fatalities from cardiovascular disease. By taking this course, participants can make a difference in saving lives in respiratory and/or cardiac emergencies.

Review

Check the correct answer.

1. The leading cause of death in the United States is—
   ☐ a. Cancer.
   ☐ b. Cardiovascular disease.
   ☐ c. Accidents.
   ☐ d. Pneumonia.

2. Advanced cardiac life support (ACLS) includes—
   ☐ a. Use of a cardiac monitor.
   ☐ b. Administration of cardiac drugs.
   ☐ c. Defibrillation.
   ☐ d. All of the above.

3. The saving of lives depends on prompt basic life support (BLS) within—
   ☐ a. 0 to 4 minutes.
   ☐ b. 5 to 6 minutes.
   ☐ c. 8 to 10 minutes.

4. The saving of lives depends on prompt advanced cardiac life support (ACLS) within—
   ☐ a. 0 to 10 minutes.
   ☐ b. 10 to 12 minutes.
   ☐ c. 12 to 14 minutes.

5. Common cardiac emergencies include cardiac arrest, angina pectoris, and—
   ☐ a. Heart attack.
   ☐ b. Stroke.
   ☐ c. Respiratory arrest.
   ☐ d. Obstructed airway.

Complete the following statement.

6. The most important priorities for the professional rescuer during the initial patient assessment are checking to see that the patient has an open _____, is _____, that the heart is beating, and that there is no severe bleeding.

Answers

1. **b.** The leading cause of death in the United States is **cardiovascular disease.**

2. **d.** Advanced cardiac life support (ACLS) includes **use of a cardiac monitor, administration of cardiac drugs,** and **defibrillation.**

3. **a.** The saving of lives depends on prompt basic life support (BLS) within **0 to 4 minutes.**

4. **a.** The saving of lives depends on prompt advanced cardiac life support (ACLS) within **0 to 10 minutes.**

5. **a.** Common cardiac emergencies include cardiac arrest, angina pectoris, and **heart attack.**

6. The most important priorities for the professional rescuer during the initial patient assessment are checking to see that the patient has an open **airway,** is **breathing,** that the heart is beating, and that there is no severe bleeding.

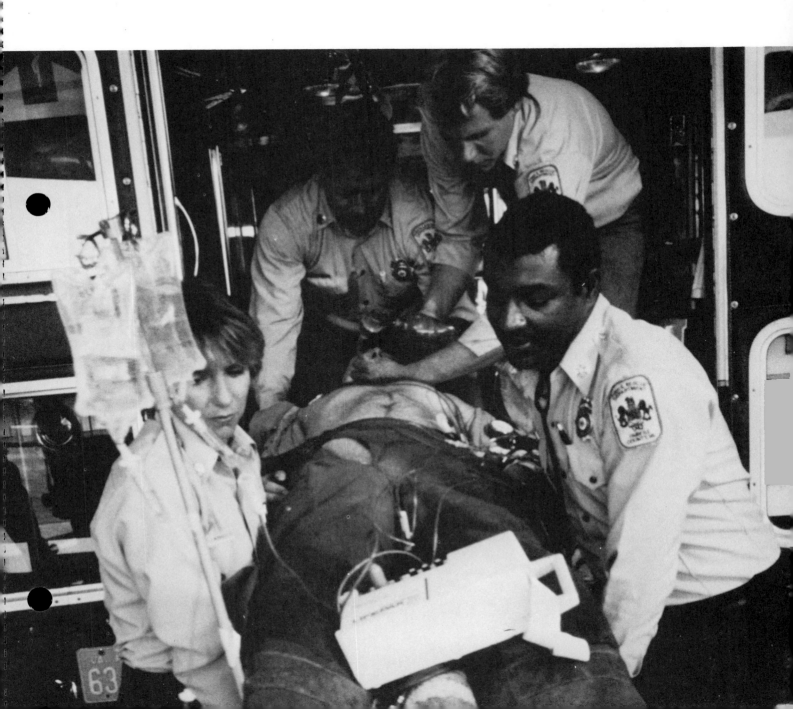

A Total Community Approach to Reducing Deaths From Cardiovascular Disease

MAIN IDEAS

1. A total community approach is needed to reduce illness and death from cardiovascular disease.
2. A total community approach includes prevention of cardiovascular disease, recognition of early warning signs of heart attack and early entry into the EMS system, and citizen CPR.
3. A community's EMS system is a vital part of a total community approach to reducing deaths from cardiovascular disease.

CHAPTER OUTLINE

I. A Total Community Approach to Saving Lives
   A. Factors leading to reduction of death rate from cardiovascular disease
   B. Prevention; recognition and EMS entry; citizen CPR
II. Emergency Cardiac Care (ECC) and the EMS System
   A. Role of an EMS system
   B. CPR is the foundation for ECC
III. The EMS System at Work
IV. Review

OBJECTIVES

1. Describe the basic parts of a total community approach to reducing deaths from cardiovascular disease.
2. Describe how an EMS system should work.

A Total Community Approach to Saving Lives

The cardiovascular disease death rate has been slowly declining since 1950. This trend suggests that several factors have helped reduce the death rate. These include—
- Greater public awareness of cardiovascular disease risk factors.
- Increased public awareness of early warning signs of heart attack and stroke.
- The beginning of CPR training for laypersons in the mid-1970s.
- The growth of EMS systems.
- Improved emergency cardiac care.
- Improved availability of coronary care.
- Better coronary care, including diagnosis, therapy, surgical techniques, and use of drugs.

A total community approach to reducing deaths from cardiovascular disease has been recommended by medical authorities as the best way to reduce deaths from cardiovascular disease. This approach, which encompasses *prevention* of cardiovascular disease as well as an emergency care response, shows the greatest promise for saving lives *(Fig. 3)*. It includes—

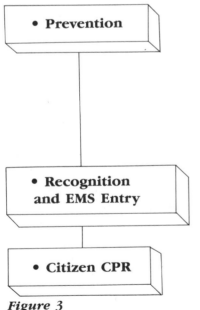

• Prevention

Stressing early recognition and control of risk factors before cardiovascular disease happens: screening for early stages of cardiovascular disease and preventing the disease from progressing, through lifestyle change and medical intervention.

• Recognition and EMS Entry

Recognizing the early warning signs of heart attack and knowing how to activate the EMS system.

• Citizen CPR

Having sufficient numbers of citizens (or laypersons) trained to provide CPR until arrival of EMS.

Figure 3

The professional rescuer is a valuable link in the total community approach to reducing cardiovascular disease. As part of the EMS system, the professional rescuer provides basic life support (BLS) until advanced cardiac life support (ACLS) is available at the scene. Prompt initiation of CPR by a professional rescuer or by a citizen, followed by ACLS, is an important component of the community effort.

Emergency Cardiac Care and the EMS System

Emergency cardiac care (ECC) includes all care necessary to deal with sudden and often life-threatening events affecting the cardiovascular system. To be effective, ECC should be an integral part of a community-wide EMS system.

An EMS system is a chain of human and physical resources brought together to provide patient care at the scene of an emergency.[3] A community EMS system is a coordinated network that links BLS, ACLS, transportation, and hospital facilities into a cohesive structure.

CPR performed by professional rescuers and laypersons is the foundation for emergency cardiac care. As discussed in Chapter 1, patient survival depends upon prompt delivery of BLS followed by ACLS. Programs that use the coordinated approach within an EMS system have been highly successful in saving lives.

The EMS System at Work

As previously described, an EMS system is a combination of human and physical resources. The professional rescuer plays an important role in linking those resources. Once activated, the system facilitates the patient's receiving continuous care in a series of stages *(Fig. 4)*.

When a medical emergency occurs, the *first stage* of emergency care begins when a citizen or a professional rescuer comes upon an accident or an emergency. After surveying the scene, conducting a primary survey, and beginning BLS if necessary, the rescuer activates the EMS system by calling or sending someone to call the community's emergency number.

The response of the EMS dispatcher is critical in the *second stage*. The dispatcher receives the emergency call and decides what equipment and personnel to send to the scene. In addition, the dispatcher may offer first aid instructions over the telephone to the caller.

In the *third stage,* emergency personnel are dispatched to the scene. This can include police officers, firefighters, emergency medical technicians (EMTs), and/or paramedics (EMT-Ps). On the way to the scene, they prepare a plan of action based on the dispatcher's information.

In the *fourth stage,* EMS personnel arrive and give emergency care at the scene. Paramedics or specially trained EMTs may need to perform defibrillation. After stabilizing the patient, they prepare him or her for transport to the hospital.

The *fifth stage* is transport to the hospital, during which emergency care continues.

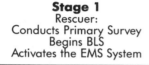
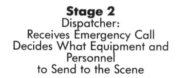
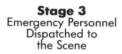
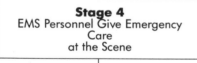
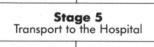
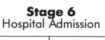

Stage 1
Rescuer:
Conducts Primary Survey
Begins BLS
Activates the EMS System

Stage 2
Dispatcher:
Receives Emergency Call
Decides What Equipment and Personnel
to Send to the Scene

Stage 3
Emergency Personnel
Dispatched to
the Scene

Stage 4
EMS Personnel Give Emergency Care
at the Scene

Stage 5
Transport to the Hospital

Stage 6
Hospital Admission

Stage 7
Hospital Recovery of the Patient

Figure 4
Stages of Care in an EMS System

The *sixth stage* begins when the patient arrives at the hospital. EMTs or paramedics provide the staff with written and oral reports of the patient's condition. In the emergency department, assessments are made of the patient's condition, and urgent needs are attended to immediately. Emergency procedures are performed if necessary.

The *seventh stage* in the process involves hospital recovery of the patient. This may include rehabilitation, therapy, and patient education.

The 1985 National Conference on Standards and Guidelines for Cardiopulmonary Resuscitation and Emergency Cardiac Care estimated that 100,000 to 200,000 lives could be saved each year in the United States if—

- More laypersons were trained in CPR.
- All professional rescuers were trained in CPR.
- All laypersons and professional rescuers knew how to activate the EMS system in the communities where they live and work.
- All communities worked to develop their EMS systems, with the potential for early defibrillation under strict medical control, so that BLS and ACLS could reach the victim quickly.

A Total Community Approach to Reducing Deaths From Cardiovascular Disease

Review

1. The following terms describe three important parts of a total community approach to reducing deaths from cardiovascular disease. In the space provided before each statement, place the word(s) from the list at the left beside the statement described.

    Citizen CPR

    Prevention

    Recognition and
      EMS Entry

    _____ Changing one's health lifestyle.

    _____ Knowing the early warning signs of a heart attack and activating the EMS system when a person shows signs of a heart attack.

    _____ Having sufficient numbers of citizens trained to provide CPR until arrival of EMS.

2. This chapter lists seven EMS operations. Number each one listed below in the order in which it is carried out.
    _____ EMS personnel give care at the scene.
    _____ Hospital recovery.
    _____ BLS started at the scene.
    _____ Patient arrives at the hospital.
    _____ Response of dispatcher.
    _____ Transport.
    _____ Emergency personnel dispatched to the scene.

Check the correct answer.

3. CPR performed by professional rescuers and laypersons is the foundation for—
   □ a. Emergency cardiac care (ECC).
   □ b. Changing one's health lifestyle.
   □ c. Recognizing a heart attack.
   □ d. Preventing cardiovascular disease.

4. A community's _____ is a combination of human and physical resources that works to provide continuous care for the patient experiencing a medical emergency.
   □ a. Emergency cardiac care committee.
   □ b. Emergency department.
   □ c. Disaster team.
   □ d. EMS system.

Answers

1. The following terms describe the three parts of a total community approach to reducing deaths from cardiovascular disease.

    Prevention: Changing one's health lifestyle.

    Recognition and EMS Entry: Knowing the early warning signs of a heart attack and activating the EMS system when a person shows signs of a heart attack.

    Citizen CPR: Having sufficient numbers of citizens trained to provide CPR until arrival of EMS.

2. The seven EMS operations are carried out in the following order:

    4. Emergency personnel give care at the scene.
    7. Hospital recovery.
    1. BLS started at the scene.
    6. Patient arrives at the hospital.
    2. Response of dispatcher.
    5. Transport.
    3. Emergency personnel dispatched to the scene.

3. a. CPR performed by professional rescuers and laypersons is the foundation for **emergency cardiac care (ECC).**

4. d. A community's **EMS system** is a combination of human and physical resources that works to provide continuous care for the patient experiencing a medical emergency.

3

The Respiratory and Circulatory Systems

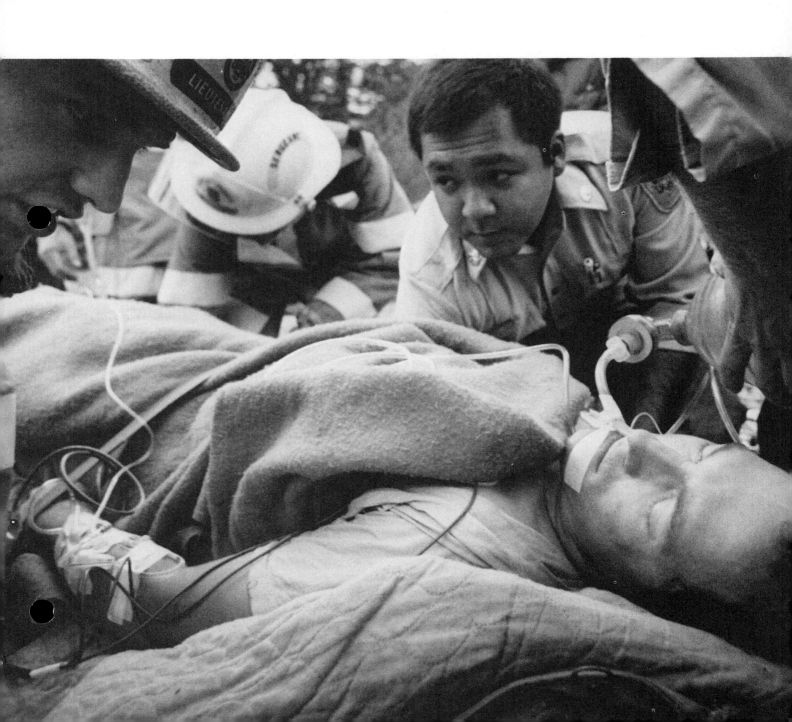

The Respiratory and Circulatory Systems

MAIN IDEAS

1. By giving CPR, the rescuer temporarily maintains the functions of the patient's respiratory and circulatory systems.
2. The respiratory and circulatory systems work together in supplying oxygen to the brain and the rest of the body.
3. CPR includes three main activities: maintaining an open Airway, and providing Breathing and Circulation (the ABCs).
4. Knowledge of how the respiratory and circulatory systems work can help the professional rescuer perform CPR.

CHAPTER OUTLINE

I. The Function of CPR
II. The ABCs of CPR:
   A. The airway
      1. Anatomy of the airway
      2. Maintaining an open airway
   B. The respiratory system
      1. The route of air and oxygen
      2. Normal breathing
   C. The circulatory system
      1. The blood vessels
      2. The heart
      3. The function of chest compressions
III. Review

OBJECTIVES

1. Identify the parts of the airway.
2. Describe how the heart and blood vessels carry oxygen to the brain and other vital organs.
3. Describe why CPR temporarily maintains the functions of the respiratory and circulatory systems during a cardiac emergency.

The Function of CPR

Each of the body's systems is composed of millions of cells, and each system plays a special role. The respiratory and circulatory systems are responsible for the most important function of the living organism: providing oxygen to the brain and other vital organs. These two systems work together as a unit, transporting oxygen to body cells and removing their waste products. CPR is an emergency procedure used when respiratory and circulatory functions have stopped.

When a person's heart stops beating, oxygen-carrying blood needs to be moved through the body to keep the brain and other organs alive. The major objective of performing CPR is to provide oxygen to the brain, heart, and other vital organs until advanced cardiac life support (ACLS) can restore normal heart and breathing action. In delivering CPR, the rescuer temporarily maintains the functions of the respiratory and circulatory systems, providing the patient with oxygen by breathing into the patient, and using external chest compressions to circulate oxygen-carrying blood through the patient's body.

The ABCs of CPR

Maintaining an open Airway and providing Breathing and Circulation are the key elements of CPR *(Fig. 5)*. The success of the rescuer giving CPR depends in part upon how quickly and effectively he or she opens the airway and provides rescue breathing and chest compressions. Knowledge of the respiratory and circulatory systems can help the professional rescuer understand how important the ABCs are.

The Airway
The airway serves as the entry point for air into the respiratory system. Air is breathed in through the mouth and nose. A clear passageway allows for a free flow of air to the lungs. The rescuer is responsible for making sure that this passageway is clear of obstruction.

As air enters through the mouth and nose *(Fig. 6)*, it passes through the **pharynx,** which is the throat. The pharynx then divides into two passageways: one for food (the **esophagus)** and one for air (the **trachea,** or windpipe). The trachea is guarded by a small valve called the **epiglottis,** which protects the opening of the trachea so that food or liquid does not enter the lungs when a person swallows. The trachea also includes the **larynx,** which is located at the top of the trachea and contains the vocal cords. The larynx is often referred to as the voice box.

PRIMARY SURVEY

AIRWAY

BREATHING

CIRCULATION

Figure 5

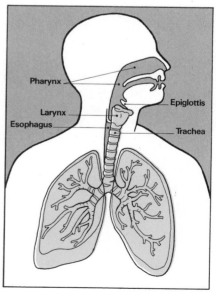

Figure 6
The Airway

21

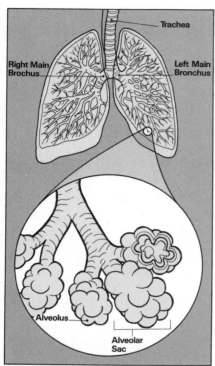

***Figure* 7**
The Airway: Lungs and Alveoli

After the air passes through the trachea, it is carried into the lungs *(Fig. 7)*. The trachea divides into two tubes called the **bronchi.** The bronchi branch out into smaller and smaller passageways. These passages end in small sacs known as **alveoli.** It is in the millions of alveoli that oxygen is transferred to the blood and exchanged for carbon dioxide that is exhaled from the body.

When the airway is blocked, oxygen cannot reach the lungs. Therefore, *the immediate opening of the airway* is the most important action for successful resuscitation. The tongue is the most common cause of airway obstruction in the unconscious patient. Maintaining an open airway is a critical skill for the professional rescuer. The steps used to open the airway are reviewed in Chapter 5. Additional methods of opening the airway are described in Chapter 7.

The Respiratory System

Air enters the respiratory system through a process known as **inhalation,** and is expelled from the system through a process known as **exhalation.** Inhaled air contains approximately 21 percent oxygen, while exhaled air contains 16 percent oxygen.

When a person breathes normally, respiration takes place automatically. The average adult breathes 12 to 20 times a minute. The body's need for oxygen is continuous because very little oxygen can be stored in the body. Rescue breathing is used when a person cannot breathe adequately on his or her own. Since the body only uses a fraction of its oxygen intake, the rescuer has enough oxygen in the exhaled air he or she breathes into the patient to support life. The steps used in performing rescue breathing are reviewed in Chapter 5.

The Circulatory System

The circulatory system is composed of the heart, blood, and blood vessels. The heart pumps blood through the blood vessels: the arteries, veins, and capillaries *(Fig. 8)*. Blood is oxygenated in the lungs and returns to the heart to be circulated through the body. From the heart, oxygen-rich blood is pumped through the arteries to the body cells. The arteries subdivide many times, ending in smaller blood vessels known as capillaries.

In the capillaries, oxygen passes from the blood into the body cells and waste gases from the body cells pass back into the blood. The blood carrying waste gases is returned to the heart through vessels known as veins, and then carried to the lungs, where the waste gases are exhaled.

The heart functions like a pump and lies directly beneath the lower half of the **sternum** (breastbone). A built-in electrical system stimulates the heart muscle to contract at regular intervals. When this electrical system breaks down, the heart cannot operate effectively. If this happens, external chest compressions are needed to keep the patient's blood circulating. The rescuer supplies these external chest compressions during CPR.

The compressions are performed directly over the heart at the lower half of the sternum. There are two major theories about how compressing the chest circulates blood. The "cardiac pump" theory says that direct compression of the heart between the sternum and the spine causes the heart to act as a pump and move blood into the arteries and through the circulatory system. In contrast, the "thoracic pump mechanism" theory states that chest compressions result in a pressure increase in the chest cavity and on the blood vessels, which causes blood to move through the system.

The volume of blood flow resulting from chest compressions is usually one-fourth to one-third of the normal flow. It is very important that chest compressions be performed properly to achieve this flow. Blood circulated to the brain as a result of chest compressions is sufficient to maintain life for a short time when combined with the oxygen supplied by properly performed rescue breathing. The steps used in combining chest compressions with rescue breathing are reviewed in Chapter 5.

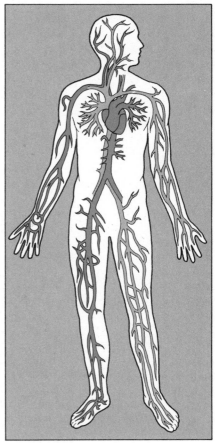

Figure 8
The Circulatory System

Review

Fill in the blanks with the correct word(s).

1. Described below are the roles of different parts of the circulatory system. Name the part or parts whose action is described.

   _____ Pumps blood through vessels of the body.

   _____ Carry blood away from the heart.

   _____ Tiny blood vessels where oxygen and waste gases are exchanged.

   _____ Carry blood back to the heart.

Check the correct answer.

2. The passageway for air leading from the throat to the lungs is known as the—
   ☐ a. Esophagus.
   ☐ b. Epiglottis.
   ☐ c. Trachea.
   ☐ d. Alveoli.

3. The _____ and circulatory systems are responsible for providing oxygen to the brain and other vital organs.
   ☐ a. Digestive.
   ☐ b. Reproductive.
   ☐ c. Nervous.
   ☐ d. Respiratory.

4. The most common cause of airway obstruction in the unconscious patient is the—
   - ☐ a. Throat.
   - ☐ b. Vocal cords.
   - ☐ c. Tongue.
   - ☐ d. Lungs.

5. Rescue breathing works because there is enough _____ in the exhaled air the rescuer breathes into the patient to support life.
   - ☐ a. Oxygen.
   - ☐ b. Nitrogen.
   - ☐ c. Carbon dioxide.
   - ☐ d. Hydrogen.

Fill in the blank with the correct word(s).

6. The circulatory system is composed of the _____, blood, and blood vessels.

Answers

1. The following parts of the circulatory system play the roles described:

    Heart: Pumps blood through vessels of the body.
    Arteries: Carry blood away from the heart.
    Capillaries: Tiny blood vessels where oxygen and waste gases are exchanged.
    Veins: Carry blood back to the heart.

2. **c.** The passageway for air leading from the throat to the lungs is known as the **trachea.**

3. **d.** The **respiratory** and circulatory systems are responsible for providing oxygen to the brain and other vital organs.

4. **c.** The most common cause of airway obstruction in the unconscious patient is the **tongue.**

5. **a.** Rescue breathing works because there is enough **oxygen** in the exhaled air the rescuer breathes into the patient to support life.

6. The circulatory system is composed of the **heart,** blood, and blood vessels.

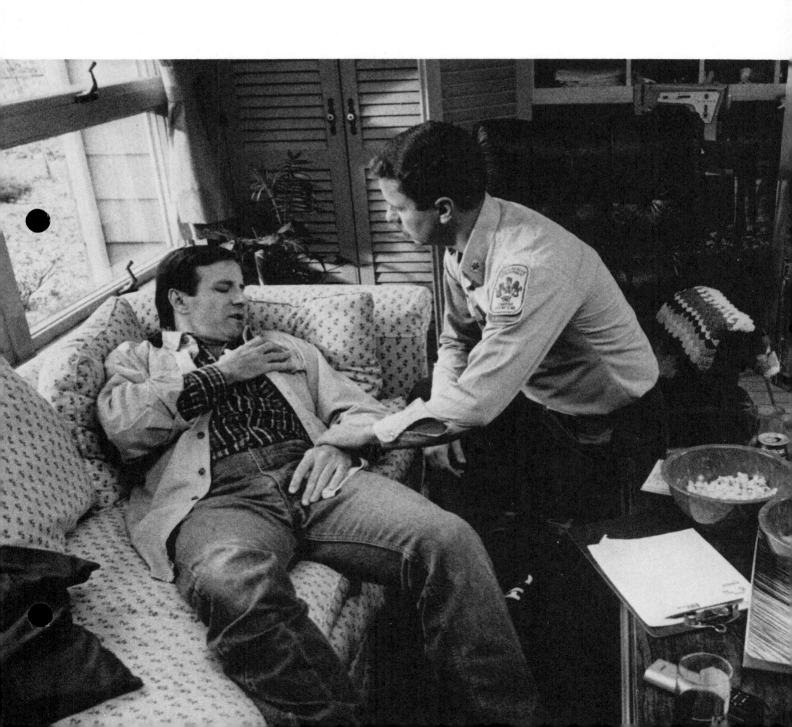

Risk Factors and Consequences of Cardiovascular Disease

MAIN IDEAS

1. The lifestyle of the professional rescuer may put him or her at high risk for cardiovascular disease.
2. Cardiovascular disease is believed to begin at an early age.
3. Risk factors for cardiovascular disease fall into three major groups.
4. The results of cardiovascular disease can lead to angina pectoris, heart attack, cardiac arrest, and stroke.
5. It is important for professional rescuers to recognize and know basic first aid for angina pectoris, heart attack, cardiac arrest, and stroke.

CHAPTER OUTLINE

   I. Risks of Cardiovascular Disease in Daily Living
  II. Risk Factors for Cardiovascular Disease That CANNOT Be Changed
 III. Risk Factors for Cardiovascular Disease That CAN Be Changed or Controlled
 IV. Contributing Risk Factors for Cardiovascular Disease
  V. How Risk Factors Contribute to Cardiovascular Disease
     A. Angina pectoris
     B. Heart attack
     C. Cardiac arrest
     D. Stroke
 VI. Review
VII. Healthy Heart I.Q.

OBJECTIVES

1. Identify heart disease risk factors that CAN and CANNOT be changed or controlled.
2. Identify the signs of angina pectoris, heart attack, cardiac arrest, and stroke.
3. Identify the actions to take for angina pectoris, heart attack, cardiac arrest, and stroke.

Reducing the Risks of Heart Disease in Daily Living

The total community approach to saving lives described in Chapter 2 indicates that the best way to prevent heart disease is to reduce risks. **Risk factors** are conditions or behaviors that increase the likelihood that a person will develop a disease. The major risk factors for cardiovascular disease include cigarette smoking, high blood pressure, and high cholesterol levels. Health habits associated with heart disease are believed to begin early in life. Since heart disease develops slowly over a long period, it is important that people understand that reducing risks should begin at an early age. Prevention of heart disease through risk reduction should become a way of life.

Some professional rescuers work in high-stress environments. Their on-the-go lifestyle can sometimes lead to poor nutritional habits. Eating "fast food" on the run can contribute to high cholesterol levels that are related to cardiovascular disease. In addition, working long hours may make it difficult to find time for a regular exercise program. Given these working conditions, the professional rescuer may want to examine carefully his or her own health behavior, and learn which risk factors can be reduced.

There are three groups of risk factors *(Fig. 9)*. The first group includes major factors that *cannot* be changed. Major factors that *can* be changed or controlled are included in the second group. The third group includes a number of factors that *contribute* to cardiovascular disease. Most of these contributing factors also can be changed or controlled.

Reducing the Risks of Heart Disease in Daily Living

Risk Factors That Cannot Be Changed
Heredity
Age
Sex

Risk Factors That Can Be Changed or Controlled
Cigarette Smoking
High Blood Pressure
High Cholesterol

Contributing Risk Factors That Can Be Changed or Controlled
Obesity
Lack of Exercise
Stress
Diabetes

Figure 9
Risk Factors for Cardiovascular Disease

Risk Factors for Cardiovascular Disease That CANNOT Be Changed

Heredity
The risk of cardiovascular disease is greater for those individuals with relatives who have had a heart attack or a stroke. Relatives include immediate family members such as parents, grandparents, brothers, and sisters.

Age
A person's risk of heart disease increases with age; the majority of deaths from cardiovascular disease occur after age 65. However, 18 percent of the individuals who die from cardiovascular disease are under the age of 65.

Sex
Men are at greater risk of developing cardiovascular disease than women. Even though the risk of heart disease increases with age

for women, the risk for men always remains higher. Nonetheless, heart disease is the leading cause of death for females.

Risk Factors for Cardiovascular Disease That CAN Be Changed or Controlled

Cigarette Smoking

According to the Surgeon General of the United States, cigarette smoking *(Fig. 10)* is the single most important cause of preventable death in this country.[4] Each puff on a cigarette causes a person's heart and arteries to react. Nicotine, just one of the many elements in cigarette smoke, plays a big role in the disease process. Nicotine constricts blood vessels, makes the heart beat faster, raises blood pressure, lowers the blood's ability to carry oxygen, and raises cholesterol levels. It has been conclusively shown that cigarette smoking contributes to cardiovascular disease.

SURGEON GENERAL'S WARNING: Quitting Smoking Now Greatly Reduces Serious Risks to Your Health.

Figure 10
Cigarette Warning Label

Hypertension (High Blood Pressure)

Hypertension, or high blood pressure, is another major risk factor that can be controlled. It is estimated that some 58 million Americans have high blood pressure. Forty million of these individuals are under the age of 65.

Blood pressure is the pressure exerted on the walls of the arteries as the blood passes through the circulatory system. Two numbers are recorded during a blood pressure measurement and are written as 120/80, for example. The first number, systolic pressure, is the pressure exerted against the artery walls when the heart contracts. The second number, diastolic pressure, is the pressure in the arteries when the heart is resting between beats.

If the arteries narrow, it becomes more difficult for the blood to pass through the circulatory system. Blood pressure in the arteries rises, and this may make the heart work harder. If the increased pressure remains above normal levels, high blood pressure develops. Over a long period of time, the heart tends to enlarge when it has to work harder than normal. High blood pressure also contributes to hardening of the arteries, which increases the possibility of stroke.

Most authorities agree that blood pressure should remain below 140/90. Hypertension can be controlled in several ways, including—

—Medication.
—Weight reduction (diet).
—Moderate exercise.
—Lowered use of alcohol.
—Lowered salt intake.
—Relaxation training.

It is important to realize that high blood pressure often goes unnoticed. Screening for hypertension can be done by local physicians, Red Cross chapters, or other health care providers.

High Cholesterol

Cholesterol is a fatty substance that is found in certain foods, and is also produced by the body. Too much cholesterol in the blood can cause a buildup of fatty deposits (**plaque**) in the arteries. This buildup can narrow and eventually block the arteries, partially or completely shutting off the blood flow, which can cause a heart attack or stroke. There is evidence that a lowered cholesterol level reduces the risk of cardiovascular disease.[5]

Recent guidelines issued by the National Heart, Lung, and Blood Institute of the National Institutes of Health recommend that all Americans over 20 years of age undergo cholesterol testing. The Institute recommends a cholesterol level of under 200 as desirable, and considers a level of over 240 as a high cholesterol level.

In most cases, cholesterol levels can be controlled by reducing the amount of saturated fat and cholesterol in the diet. Saturated fats are found in meats, animal fats, dairy products, some vegetable oils (palm oil and coconut oil), shortening, and bakery goods. Foods highest in saturated fats and cholesterol include eggs, cheese, butter, whole milk, fatty meats, and fried foods.

A program of regular exercise and a diet that is low in saturated fats and cholesterol can help lower cholesterol levels. Foods low in saturated fats and cholesterol include fresh fruits and vegetables, grains and cereals, low-fat dairy products, and certain vegetable oils (sunflower, safflower, sesame, corn, and soybean). If necessary, a physician can prescribe medication to help lower very high cholesterol levels.

The Contributing Risk Factors for Cardiovascular Disease That Can Be Changed or Controlled

Obesity

A person is considered obese if he or she is 20 percent over-weight according to height-weight tables *(Fig. 11)*. (Because of variations in individual frame size, height-weight tables may not indicate the correct weight range for all people.) Obese individuals are at greater risk of cardiovascular disease mainly because they tend to have high blood pressure and high cholesterol levels. Extra weight also causes the heart muscle and its network of blood vessels to work harder.

METROPOLITAN HEIGHT AND WEIGHT TABLES

MEN					WOMEN				
Height		Small	Medium	Large		Height	Small	Medium	Large
Feet	Inches	Frame	Frame	Frame	Feet	Inches	Frame	Frame	Frame
5	2	128-134	131-141	138-150	4	10	102-111	109-121	118-131
5	3	130-136	133-143	140-153	4	11	103-113	111-123	120-134
5	4	132-138	135-145	142-156	5	0	104-115	113-126	122-137
5	5	134-140	137-148	144-160	5	1	106-118	115-129	125-140
5	6	136-142	139-151	146-164	5	2	108-121	118-132	128-143
5	7	138-145	142-154	149-168	5	3	111-124	121-135	131-147
5	8	140-148	145-157	152-172	5	4	114-127	124-138	134-151
5	9	142-151	148-160	155-176	5	5	117-130	127-141	137-155
5	10	144-154	151-163	158-180	5	6	120-133	130-144	140-159
5	11	146-157	154-166	161-184	5	7	123-136	133-147	143-163
6	0	149-160	157-170	164-188	5	8	126-139	136-150	146-167
6	1	152-164	160-174	168-192	5	9	129-142	139-153	149-170
6	2	155-168	164-178	172-197	5	10	132-145	142-156	152-173
6	3	158-172	167-182	176-202	5	11	135-148	145-159	155-176
6	4	162-176	171-187	181-207	6	0	138-151	148-162	158-179

Weights at ages 25-59 based on lowest mortality. Weight in pounds according to frame (in indoor clothing weighing 5 lbs. for men and 3 lbs. for women; shoes with 1'' heels).

Height and Weight Tables Courtesy Statistical Bulletin, *Metropolitan Life Insurance Company, 1983*

Figure 11

Lack of Exercise

Individuals who do not exercise usually have a faster heart rate and a smaller capillary network than people who do exercise regularly. A greater network of capillaries allows for more efficient transfer of oxygen to the cells. Physically active individuals who follow a regular plan of aerobic exercise (walking, running, cycling, swimming, or aerobic dance) suffer fewer heart attacks than people who do not exercise. A program of regular exercise strengthens the heart and blood vessels. It also increases the ability of the heart and blood vessels to circulate blood efficiently.

Stress

Stress causes physical, emotional, and behavioral reactions, although people react to stress differently. Some personalities seem to go through life more relaxed than others. Some individuals are more seriously affected by stressful situations. The body may react to stress by causing blood vessels to constrict, increasing blood pressure, and stimulating the liver to produce more cholesterol.

Diabetes

Diabetes is a complex disease in which the body is unable to turn blood sugars (from food) into energy. This occurs when there is a decrease in the production or activity of the hormone insulin; body cells cannot use blood sugar unless insulin is present. Some individuals develop diabetes in childhood, but most diabetics develop the disease in their 50s or 60s.

Diabetics are at increased risk of cardiovascular disease. Approximately 75 percent of the deaths occurring in diabetics are caused by some form of cardiovascular disease. Although the relationship between cardiovascular disease and diabetes is not completely understood, it is known that diabetes can damage both small and large blood vessels, and that diabetics are more likely to experience other risk factors associated with cardiovascular disease. These risk factors include hypertension, high cholesterol levels, and obesity.

Note: Specific questions about any of the information included in these risk factors should be referred to a health care provider.

How Risk Factors Contribute to Cardiovascular Disease

Health habits associated with cardiovascular disease can begin at an early age. A person who does not recognize and reduce his or her risk of cardiovascular disease may find that, eventually, the effects of risk factors take their toll. Over a period of years, plaque gradually builds up on the walls of the arteries. This is a condition known as **atherosclerosis.** As plaque builds up, the arteries narrow. These arteries become harder and thicker, and the opening for blood flow becomes smaller. Thus, the flow of blood through the arteries becomes partially or completely blocked *(Fig. 12),* leading to angina pectoris, heart attack **(myocardial infarction),** cardiac arrest, or stroke.

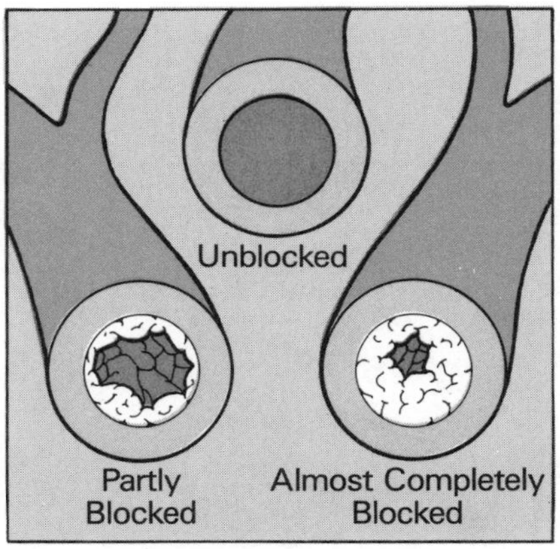

Figure 12
Blocked Arteries

Recognition and Emergency Care for Angina Pectoris, Heart Attack, Cardiac Arrest, and Stroke

Angina Pectoris

Angina pectoris, often called angina, is a condition that develops when the heart needs more oxygen than it is able to get. This lack of oxygen results in a constricting chest pain that may spread to the neck, jaw, and arms. This pain is usually less severe than that of a heart attack, and it usually lasts between 2 and 10 minutes.

The greatest contributing factor to angina is **coronary atherosclerosis,** which narrows the arteries and restricts circulation to the heart. Other causes include strenuous activity, which places great oxygen demands on the heart and increases both the heart rate and blood pressure; emotional stress; and temperature extremes. Angina can usually be relieved by resting and/or taking medication **(nitroglycerin).**

It is difficult to determine if a patient with an unknown heart disease history is experiencing angina or a heart attack. For this reason, appropriate emergency medical care for angina should follow the steps outlined for emergency care for heart attack.

Heart Attack (Myocardial Infarction)

A heart attack occurs when the oxygen supply to the heart muscle **(myocardium)** is cut off for a prolonged period of time. This cutoff results from a reduced blood supply due to severe narrowing or complete blockage of a diseased artery. The result is death (infarction) of the affected part of the heart.

The most significant signal of a heart attack is chest discomfort or pain that ranges from uncomfortable, squeezing pressure to unbearable crushing or stabbing pain. This pain may be continuous, or it may come and go. The pain is usually in the center of the chest, underneath the breastbone. It may spread to both shoulders, arms, neck, jaw, or back *(Fig. 13).* Additional signals include shortness of breath, sweating, and nausea. Unlike the pain of angina pectoris, the pain associated with a heart attack usually lasts longer than 10 minutes and is not relieved by rest and/or nitroglycerin. *Note:* Sometimes victims of heart attack have no symptoms and experience no pain.

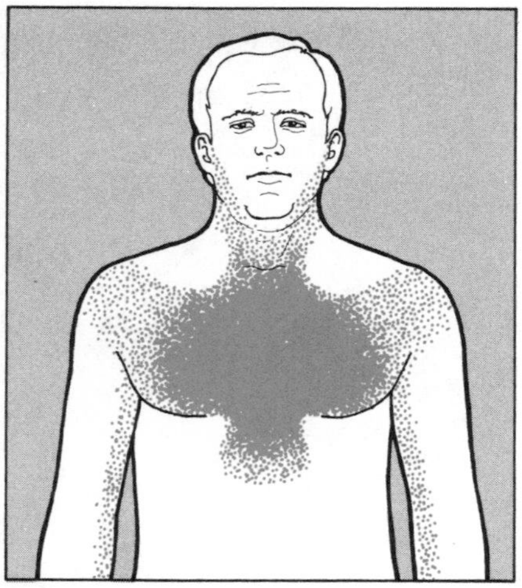

The emergency care for both heart attack and angina begins with recognition of the signals of heart attack. The initial care is to have the patient stop what he or she is doing and rest in a comfortable position that allows the patient to breathe easily. The rescuer should ask the patient if he or she has a history of heart disease, and contact the EMS system. If the patient has a known history of heart disease and is taking nitroglycerin, the rescuer should assist the patient in taking his or her medication. The rescuer should continue to reassure and calm the patient.

Figure 13
Areas for Heart Attack Pain

Cardiac Arrest

Cardiac arrest, or sudden cardiac death, causes breathing and circulation to cease abruptly. It may occur before any signal of a heart attack. Coronary heart disease is the most common cause of cardiac arrest. Other factors, such as respiratory arrest, shock, chest trauma, and disturbance of normal cardiac rhythm, also are associated with cardiac arrest.

One disturbance in cardiac rhythm that often causes cardiac arrest is **ventricular fibrillation.** It is caused by electrical interference from the injured area of the heart. This chaotic, uncoordinated electrical activity keeps the heart from pumping effectively.

Although CPR can keep a victim's brain alive, cardiac arrest due to ventricular fibrillation can seldom be reversed without electrical defibrillation. **Defibrillation** is the application of an external electric shock to the victim's heart that re-establishes the heart's regular electrical activity, producing an effective heartbeat. Prompt application of CPR and successful defibrillation will greatly increase the patient's chance for survival.

Stroke

A stroke, or **cerebral vascular accident,** occurs when blood flow to the brain is interrupted long enough to cause damage. Atherosclerosis not only obstructs arteries in the heart, but also affects arteries carrying oxygen-rich blood to the brain. A stroke occurs if an artery to the brain is blocked or ruptures.

There are three causes of stroke. Most commonly, a clot forms in an artery in the brain **(cerebral thrombosis) (Fig. 14).** Clotting can also occur elsewhere in the body and be carried by the bloodstream to the arteries in the brain **(cerebral embolism).**

A second cause of stroke occurs when an artery in the brain ruptures or hemorrhages, resulting in an insufficient oxygen supply to the brain tissues and nerves. Hemorrhage may be caused by head injury, high blood pressure, a weak spot in the cerebral arteries **(aneurysm),** or atherosclerosis.

The third cause of stroke is compression of an artery in the brain, which results in restricted blood flow. A brain tumor is a likely cause of compression.

The general signals of stroke include weakness or numbness of the face, arm, or leg, often on only one side. Other possible signals include difficulty speaking, dimmed vision, or loss of vision in one eye, double vision, dizziness, confusion, loss of consciousness, and/or severe headache.

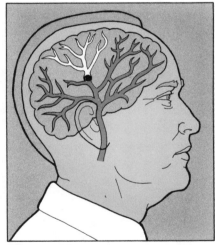

Figure 14
Stroke

When providing emergency care for stroke, the professional rescuer should make the victim stop what he or she is doing and rest. The EMS system should be contacted immediately. The patient should not eat or drink anything. If the patient becomes unconscious or begins to vomit, he or she should be turned onto the side, with the paralyzed side down, so that secretions can drain from the mouth. If respiratory and/or cardiac arrest occur, the rescuer must begin basic life support immediately.

Risk Factors and Consequences of Cardiovascular Disease

Review

1. Below is a list of risk factors for cardiovascular disease. Some of these risk factors can be changed or controlled. Others cannot. Next to each risk factor, write **yes** if it can be changed or controlled.

Risk Factor	Can Be Changed or Controlled
1. Age	_____
2. High cholesterol	_____
3. Cigarette smoking	_____
4. Heredity	_____
5. Hypertension	_____
6. Lack of exercise	_____
7. Obesity	_____
8. Stress	_____
9. Diabetes	_____

2. In the left column is a list of signals and actions for angina, heart attack, cardiac arrest, and stroke. Identify each by writing one of the following on the blank line next to each statement: angina, heart attack, cardiac arrest, or stroke.

1. Often caused by ventricular fibrillation, a chaotic and uncoordinated electrical activity of the heart. _____

2. Signals include weakness or numbness of the face, arm, or leg, often only on one side. _____

3. Usually relieved by resting and/or taking medication. _____

4. Chest discomfort or pain that may spread to shoulders, arms, neck, jaw, or back. Pain may or may not be continuous and usually lasts longer than 10 minutes. _____

5. If the patient becomes unconscious or begins to vomit, the patient is turned onto his or her side, with paralyzed side down, so that secretions can drain from the mouth. _____

6. Constricting chest pain that usually lasts 2 to 10 minutes. _____

7. Causes breathing and circulation to cease abruptly. _____

8. Occurs when an artery to the brain is blocked or ruptures. _____

Risk Factors and Consequences of Cardiovascular Disease

Answers

1. The following risk factors can be changed or controlled:
   2. **High cholesterol**
   3. **Cigarette smoking**
   5. **Hypertension**
   6. **Lack of exercise**
   7. **Obesity**
   8. **Stress**
   9. **Diabetes**

2. In the left column is a list of signals and actions for angina, heart attack, cardiac arrest, and stroke. Identify each by writing one of the following on the blank line next to each statement: angina, heart attack, cardiac arrest, and stroke.

   1. Often caused by ventricular fibrillation, a chaotic and uncoordinated electrical activity of the heart. **Cardiac arrest**

   2. Signals include weakness or numbness of the face, arm, or leg, often only on one side. **Stroke**

   3. Usually relieved by resting and/or taking medication. **Angina**

   4. Chest discomfort or pain that may spread to shoulders, arms, neck, jaw, or back. Pain may be or may not be continuous and usually lasts longer than 10 minutes. **Heart attack**

   5. If the patient becomes unconscious or begins to vomit, the patient is turned onto his or her side, with paralyzed side down, so that secretions can drain from the mouth. **Stroke**

   6. Constricting chest pain that usually lasts 2 to 10 minutes. **Angina**

   7. Causes breathing and circulation to cease abruptly. **Cardiac arrest**

   8. Occurs when an artery to the brain is blocked or ruptures. **Stroke**

test your HEALTHY HEART I.Q.

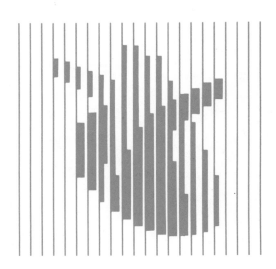

Prepared by the National Heart, Lung, and Blood Institute

The "Healthy Heart I.Q." was developed by the National Heart, Lung, and Blood Institute to help people test their knowledge of cardiovascular disease and learn what they can do to reduce some of the risks of developing it. Because prevention is part of the total community approach to reducing deaths from cardiovascular disease, the American Red Cross has included this questionnaire for course participants.

Although the test is not required, responding to the questions and reading the answers that follow is a good way for participants to assess their knowledge of risk factors. They may then want to consider whether their own health lifestyle needs to be modified.

	TRUE	FALSE
1. The three most important heart disease risk factors that you *can do something about* are: high blood pressure, smoking, and elevated blood cholesterol.	☐	☐
2. A heart attack or stroke is often the first symptom of high blood pressure and/or elevated blood cholesterol.	☐	☐
3. People with high blood pressure are generally nervous and tense people.	☐	☐
4. A blood pressure of 140/90 or more is generally considered to be high.	☐	☐
5. High blood pressure is even more of a problem among blacks than it is among whites.	☐	☐

Risk Factors and Consequences of Cardiovascular Disease

	TRUE	FALSE
6. It is only a scientific theory that elevated blood cholesterol is related to heart disease.	☐	☐
7. Dietary cholesterol is found only in animal foods.	☐	☐
8. The most effective dietary way to lower the level of your blood cholesterol is by eating less cholesterol.	☐	☐
9. A food product in your grocery store that is labeled "no cholesterol" is a safe choice for people with elevated cholesterol levels.	☐	☐
10. Cigarette smoking by itself will increase your risk of heart attack.	☐	☐
11. In addition to the large number of cancer and heart disease deaths that result from smoking, more than 90 percent of all emphysema deaths are due to smoking.	☐	☐
12. People who quit smoking reduce their chances of developing heart disease.	☐	☐
13. Heart disease is the number two killer of women in the United States.	☐	☐
14. Physical inactivity is related to heart disease.	☐	☐

Answers to the Healthy Heart I.Q. Test

1. **True.** Though there are other risk factors that you cannot change, such as family history and age, the three major risk factors that you *can* change are *high blood pressure, smoking, and elevated blood cholesterol.* Someone who has all three of these risk factors is about *eight times* as likely to develop heart disease as someone who has none of them.

2. **True.** A person with high blood pressure or elevated blood cholesterol may feel fine and look great; there are often no signs at all that might signal these conditions until a heart attack or stroke occurs. To find out if you have elevated blood cholesterol or high blood pressure, you should be tested by a doctor, nurse, or other qualified health professional. The blood cholesterol test currently requires a laboratory analysis of a sample of your blood.

3. **False.** High blood pressure does not mean that a person is nervous or tense. It means that the blood flowing through your body is pressing against your artery walls too strongly. Calm and relaxed people can have high blood pressure.

4. **True.** The higher your blood pressure is, the higher your risk of developing heart disease or having a stroke. To reduce high blood pressure—that is 140/90 or higher (either number)—it must be *treated and controlled.* If you have high blood pressure, follow your doctor's advice: get and keep your weight down to normal; decrease your consumption of sodium—not only table salt, but also foods with a high sodium content such as some snack and processed foods; and remember to take your medicine if it is prescribed.

5. **True.** While high blood pressure affects more than 28 out of every 100 white adults, it affects more than 38 out of every 100 black adults. Also, high blood pressure is generally more severe among blacks than whites.

6. **False.** Scientific studies have shown that people with high blood cholesterol are more likely to develop heart disease than people with lower levels of blood cholesterol. People with a blood cholesterol over 265 mg/dl (milligrams per deciliter of blood) may have four times the risk of developing heart disease as those with a level of 190 mg/dl or lower. It also has been shown that people who have elevated blood cholesterol and reduce it also reduce their risk of having a heart attack.

7. **True.** Dietary cholesterol is never found in foods from plants. All meat, poultry, fish, and butterfat contain cholesterol; the richest sources are liver, brains, kidneys, and egg yolks.

8. **False.** Reducing the amount of cholesterol in your diet is clearly important; however, *eating less saturated fat* would probably be the more effective dietary means of lowering your blood cholesterol levels, along with eating less cholesterol and substituting polyunsaturated fat whenever possible for saturated fat. Saturated fat (found in meats, dairy products such as whole milk, cream, ice cream, cheese, butter, and certain cooking fats like shortening) contribute greatly to the raising of blood cholesterol. To reduce your consumption of saturated fat, you should choose lean meats, poultry, or fish; trim excess fat off meats before cooking; broil, bake, or boil rather than fry; and use skim or low-fat dairy products.

9. **False.** A product can contain no cholesterol and still be *high in saturated fat*—which will *raise* your blood cholesterol. Examples are commercial baked foods made with coconut oil, palm oil, or a heavily hydrogenated vegetable oil. As you shop, be sure to check the labels on food products. You will often find a listing of the amounts of saturated and polyunsaturated fat contained in the product. Your best choice is a product that contains more polyunsaturated fat than saturated fat; *polyunsaturated fat* will *lower* your blood cholesterol. Vegetable oils that are high in polyunsaturated fat include safflower, sunflower, corn, and soybean oil.

   Remember, though, that *all* fats are a rich source of calories, and for people who are overweight, it is desirable to consume fewer calories and less fat of all kinds.

10. **True.** Smoking is a definite and strong risk factor for heart disease. The heart disease death rate among smokers is 70 percent greater than that of nonsmokers. Heavy smokers are, of course, at even greater risk, and those smokers with elevated blood cholesterol or high blood pressure increase their chances of heart disease dramatically.

11. **True.** Emphysema, a lung disease that makes breathing difficult and often leads to death, would be almost eliminated if people did not smoke.

12. **True.** Absolutely. Smokers can and do reduce their risk of coronary heart disease and early death when they quit smoking. In one major study, cigarette smokers who quit smoking had a risk of heart disease death that was about one-half (54 percent) that of those who did not quit.

13. **False.** It is the number one killer. Of the 750,000 Americans who die each year of heart disease, 350,000 are women. In addition, almost 100,000 women die each year of stroke.

14. **True.** People who are inactive tend to have more heart disease than people who are physically active. Regular brisk and sustained exercise improves overall conditioning. It can often help reduce blood pressure levels and also help people lose excess weight and lower blood cholesterol. In addition, there are reports which suggest that smokers who exercise are more likely to give up smoking. Finally, regular aerobic exercise can improve the way you look and feel.

Prepared by the U.S. Department of Health and Human Services, Public Health Service, National Institutes of Health, July 1985. Reprinted with permission.

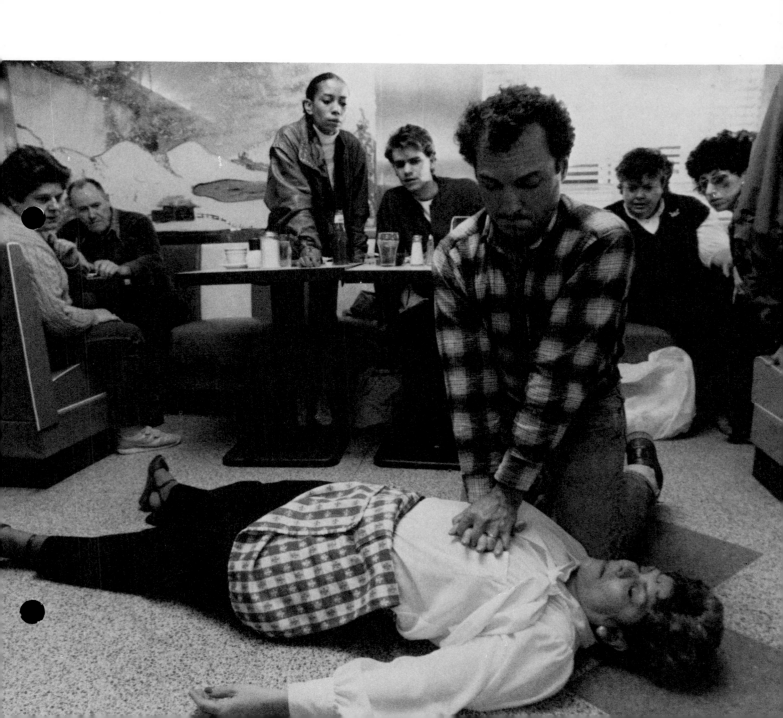

MAIN IDEAS

1. Before taking the professional rescuer course, a participant must demonstrate competency in basic CPR skills.
2. The fundamental skills reviewed in this chapter include the emergency action principles and the skills needed to give basic life support (BLS) to adults, children, and infants.

CHAPTER OUTLINE

I. Purpose of the Review
II. Reviewing the Emergency Action Principles
III. Reviewing Fundamental Skills
   A. Preventing disease transmission
   B. One-rescuer CPR
      1. Adult
      2. Child
      3. Infant
   C. Obstructed airway management
      1. Conscious adult
      2. Conscious infant
      3. Unconscious adult
      4. Unconscious infant

OBJECTIVES

1. Review major concepts of the emergency action principles.
2. Demonstrate proficiency in the fundamental skills of CPR.

Purpose of the Review

The new skills taught in the professional rescuer course build on CPR skills that participants have already learned. For this reason, individuals need to demonstrate the ability to perform the fundamental CPR skills.

The fundamental skills review is self-paced in order to accommodate the varied backgrounds of individuals enrolled in the course. Participants have the opportunity to progress through the review at their own speed. Participants who have had considerable practice and experience in performing the fundamental skills may complete the review in a short period of time. The review includes the following areas:

I. Emergency Action Principles

II. One-rescuer CPR
   A. Adult
   B. Child
   C. Infant

III. Obstructed Airway Management
   A. Conscious adult
   B. Conscious infant
   C. Unconscious adult
   D. Unconscious infant

Reviewing the Fundamentals: The Emergency Action Principles

Material in this section is covered in the review video. The written section that follows may be used by participants who wish to review the emergency action principles outside the classroom.

In every emergency, there are standard guidelines that the professional rescuer must follow. These guidelines are known as the "emergency action principles." The same basic steps are followed consistently in order to protect the safety of both patient and rescuer. The emergency action principles include—

1. Surveying the scene.
2. Performing a primary survey of the patient.
3. Activating the EMS system (if not already done).
4. Performing a secondary survey of the patient.

Each of the four steps is carried out in the order in which it is listed. By following this action plan, the professional rescuer determines whether or not it is necessary to provide basic life support (BLS).

Note: Because this course is offered to a broad audience of professional rescuers, the experience and professional responsibilities of people enrolled in the course will vary greatly. In reviewing the emergency action principles, participants need to consider their roles as part of the EMS system. For example, in CPR courses designed for and taught to the lay rescuer, the rescuer at the scene of an emergency is instructed to call the EMS system as one of the emergency action principles.

As professional rescuers, however, many of the people taking this course will arrive on the scene as *part* of the EMS system.

In another example, a police officer is often dispatched to an accident by the EMS dispatcher at the same time an ambulance is sent. The officer would not call the EMS to activate the system; rather, he or she would usually call the EMS dispatcher to confirm that BLS had been started and/or that ACLS was needed at the scene.

On the other hand, if a lifeguard or a park ranger on the job came upon an emergency, he or she *would* take the necessary action to activate the EMS system.

Identification and Permission

It is important that the rescuer identify him or herself as a professional rescuer trained in emergency care. This helps reassure patients and bystanders.

It is also important to ask permission to assist a conscious person. Legally, the person must consent to an offer of help before the professional rescuer can give assistance. (The law assumes that an unconscious person would give consent.) Consent should also be obtained from the parent or guardian of individuals who are infants, children, or mentally incompetent. If a parent or guardian is not available, emergency care to maintain life may be given without consent. The Appendix provides clarifying information on the obligation to provide CPR, Good Samaritan laws, and issues of liability.

Directions for the Participant: Reviewing Fundamental Skills

When possible, it is recommended that participants review and practice fundamental CPR skills before attending this session. During the fundamental skills review session, participants must demonstrate their ability to perform the skills correctly before beginning the next section of the workbook. After watching the video, participants begin working on the skills with a partner. This includes the following steps:

1. **View** the video demonstration of the skill.
2. **Read** the description of the skill on the skill checklist.

3. **Practice** the skill with a partner.
   a. One partner reads the steps on the skill checklist aloud, while the other partner performs the steps.
   b. The participant who is observing corrects any practice errors by telling his or her partner the *correct* changes needed. Direct statements of how the skill should be performed provide the practicing participant with immediate clues for corrections.
4. **Review** the video demonstration of the skill at any time by replaying the videocassette when needed. A quick look at how the skill is performed often saves time and energy, and provides the participant with the visual clues needed for continued progress.
5. The practicing partner **requests** a final skill check from the observing partner when he or she feels able to perform the skill correctly without prompting. The observing partner checks off each step in the Partner Check (PC) column on the skill checklist.
6. **Request** a final skill check from the instructor when one or both partners believe they are ready to demonstrate the skill as it should be performed. Participants needing more practice time should continue practicing that skill before moving to the next skill in the sequence.

To complete the fundamental skills review, the participant must get the instructor's signature on the bottom of each skill checklist to document correct performance of the skills. The participant is then ready to proceed with learning the professional rescuer skills in Part II of this course.

At the conclusion of the professional rescuer course, participants are required to pass a written test.

Health Precautions for Using the CPR Manikins

Participants practice review skills on manikins during Part I of this course, and practice new professional rescuer skills on manikins in Part II. Therefore, it is essential for them to read the following guidelines.

Red Cross chapters have been given health precautions and guidelines for using and cleaning the manikins used in CPR training. When these guidelines are followed, there is no known risk of disease transmission. Participants are asked to read this information.

Preventing Disease Transmission

Since the beginning of citizen training in CPR (cardiopulmonary resuscitation), the American Red Cross and the American Heart Association have trained more than 50 million people. According to the Centers for Disease Control (CDC), there has never been a reported case of any infectious disease transmitted through the use of CPR manikins. This may be partially due to the standards followed in the manikin decontamination procedure.

Additionally, the following is asked of course participants. Participants should not use the training manikin:

- If they have any cuts or sores on hands, head, face, lips, or mouth (for example, cold sores).
- If they are known to be seropositive for hepatitis B surface antigen (ABsAg).
- If they have any respiratory infections, such as a cold or a sore throat.
- If they are infected by the AIDS (acquired immune deficiency syndrome) virus or have AIDS.
- If they have recently been exposed to or are showing symptoms of any infectious disease.

To protect themselves and other participants from infection, participants should do the following:

- Wash hands thoroughly before working with the manikins.
- Refrain from eating, drinking, or using tobacco products immediately before or during manikin use.
- Before using the manikin, dry the manikin's face with a clean gauze pad. Next, vigorously wipe the entire face of the manikin and the inside of the mouth with a clean gauze pad soaked with a solution of sodium hypochlorite (household bleach and water) or rubbing alcohol. Place the wet pad over the manikin's mouth and nose and wait at least 30 seconds before wiping the face dry with a clean gauze pad.
- When practicing what to do for an obstructed airway, simulate (pretend to do) the finger sweep.
- When practicing two-rescuer CPR, simulate blowing into the manikin when taking over ventilation.

Additional, detailed guidelines on disease transmission can be found in the introduction to Part II on page 62 of this workbook.

Protecting Participants From Injury

CPR requires strenuous activity. Any participant who has a medical condition or disability that prevents him or her from taking part in the practice sessions should advise the instructor.

Protecting Manikins From Damage

In order to protect the manikins from damage, participants should do the following before beginning to practice:

- Remove pens and pencils from pockets.
- Remove all jewelry.
- Remove lipstick and excess makeup.
- Remove chewing gum and candy from mouths.

Review and Fundamental Skills Checklists

Skill Checklist: One-rescuer CPR (Adult)

Critical Skill	Steps	PC	IC
Check for Unresponsiveness	Tap or gently shake patient. Shout, "Are you OK?"		
Shout for Help	Shout for help to attract another person's attention.		
Position the Patient	Roll patient onto back if necessary: place one hand on patient's shoulder and other hand on patient's hip, and roll patient toward you as a unit. As you roll patient, support back of head and neck.		
Open the Airway	Using the head-tilt/chin-lift method, tilt head and lift jaw.		
Check for Breathlessness	Maintain open airway. Look at chest; listen and feel for breathing for 3 to 5 seconds.		
Give 2 Full Breaths	Maintain open airway. Pinch nose shut. Give 2 full breaths at the rate of 1 to 1½ seconds per breath. Observe chest rise and fall; listen and feel for escaping air.		
Check for Pulse	Feel for carotid pulse for 5 to 10 seconds.		
Phone the EMS System for Help	Tell someone to call for an ambulance.		
Locate Compression Position	Slide middle and index fingers of hand nearest patient's legs up the rib cage and locate "notch" at lower end of patient's breastbone. Place heel of hand nearest patient's head on breastbone next to index finger of hand used to find "notch." Place heel of hand used to locate "notch" directly on top of heel of other hand.		
Give 15 Compressions	Position shoulders over hands with elbows locked and arms straight. Compress breastbone 1½ to 2 inches at a rate of 80 to 100 compressions per minute.		
Give 2 Full Breaths	Maintain open airway. Pinch nose shut. Give 2 full breaths at the rate of 1 to 1½ seconds per breath. Observe chest rise and fall; listen and feel for escaping air.		
Do Compression/ Breathing Cycles	Do 4 cycles of 15 compressions and 2 breaths.		
Recheck Pulse	Feel for carotid pulse for 5 seconds.		
Give 2 Full Breaths	If no pulse, maintain open airway, pinch nose shut, and give 2 full breaths at the rate of 1 to 1½ seconds per breath. Observe chest rise and fall; listen and feel for escaping air.		
Continue Compression/ Breathing Cycles	Continue cycles of 15 compressions and 2 breaths. Recheck pulse every few minutes.		
Decision Making	Based on the information the instructor gives, make a decision about what to do next, and continue giving the appropriate care.		

Final Instructor Check _____

Skill Checklist: One-rescuer CPR (Child)

Critical Skill	Steps	PC	IC
Check for Unresponsiveness	Tap or gently shake child's shoulder. Shout, "Are you OK?"		
Shout for Help	Shout for help to attract another person's attention.		
Position the Child	Roll child onto back if necessary, supporting back of head and neck.		
Open the Airway	Using the head-tilt/chin-lift method, tilt the head gently back into the neutral-plus position; lift chin.		
Check for Breathlessness	Maintain open airway. Look at chest and abdomen; listen and feel for breathing for 3 to 5 seconds.		
Give 2 Slow Breaths	Give 2 slow breaths at the rate of 1 to 1½ seconds per breath.		
Check for Pulse	Feel for carotid pulse for 5 to 10 seconds.		
Phone the EMS System for Help	Tell someone to call for an ambulance.		
Locate Compression Position	Maintain head-tilt with hand on forehead. Slide middle finger of hand nearest child's legs up the rib cage to locate "notch" at lower end of breastbone. Place middle finger in "notch" and index finger next to it on the lower end of the breastbone. Look at where your index finger is placed, then lift fingers off breastbone. Place heel of same hand on the breastbone immediately above where index finger was placed.		
Give 5 Compressions	Compress breastbone 1 to 1½ inches at a rate of 80 to 100 compressions per minute. Use one hand only.		
Give 1 Slow Breath	Give 1 slow breath at the rate of 1 to 1½ seconds per breath.		
Do Compression/ Breathing Cycles	Maintain head-tilt with hand on forehead. Visually landmark compression position. Return hand doing chin-lift directly to compression position. Do 10 cycles of 5 compressions and 1 breath.		
Recheck Pulse	Feel for carotid pulse for 5 seconds.		
Give 1 Slow Breath	If no pulse, maintain open airway, pinch nose shut, and give 1 slow breath at the rate of 1 to 1½ seconds per breath. Observe chest rise and fall; listen and feel for escaping air.		
Continue Compression/ Breathing Cycles	Continue cycles of 5 compressions and 1 breath. Recheck pulse every few minutes.		
Decision Making	Based on the information the instructor gives, make a decision about what to do next, and continue giving the appropriate care.		

Final Instructor Check _____

Review and Fundamental Skills Checklists

Skill Checklist: CPR (Infant)

Critical Skill	Steps	PC	IC
Check for Unresponsiveness	Tap or gently shake infant's shoulder.		
Shout for Help	Shout for help to attract another person's attention.		
Position the Infant	Roll infant onto back if necessary, supporting back of head and neck.		
Open the Airway	Using the head-tilt/chin-lift method, gently tilt the head back into the neutral position; lift chin.		
Check for Breathlessness	Maintain open airway. Look at chest and abdomen; listen and feel for breathing for 3 to 5 seconds.		
Give 2 Slow Breaths	Give 2 slow breaths at the rate of 1 to 1½ seconds per breath. Breathe into infant's mouth and nose.		
Check for Pulse	Feel for brachial pulse for 5 to 10 seconds.		
Phone the EMS System for Help	Tell someone to call for an ambulance.		
Locate Compression Position	Maintain head-tilt with hand on forehead. Place pad of index finger on infant's breastbone just below the imaginary line connecting the nipples. Place pads of the middle and ring fingers next to index finger, then raise index finger. Pads of fingers should run down the length of the breastbone. If you feel the notch at the end of the infant's breastbone, move your fingers up the breastbone slightly.		
Give 5 Compressions	Compress breastbone ½ to 1 inch at a rate of at least 100 compressions per minute.		
Give 1 Slow Breath	Stop compressions; maintain finger position on chest. Maintain head-tilt with hand on forehead. Give 1 slow breath at a rate of 1 to 1½ seconds per breath. Observe chest rise and fall; listen and feel for escaping air. If chest does not rise, use hand on chest to perform chin-lift.		
Do Compression/ Breathing Cycles	Do 10 cycles of 5 compressions and 1 breath.		
Recheck Pulse	Feel for brachial pulse for 5 seconds with hand that was giving compressions.		
Give 1 Slow Breath	Return hand to chest; locate compression position. Give 1 slow breath at the rate of 1 to 1½ seconds per breath. If chest does not rise, use hand on chest to perform chin-lift.		
Continue Compression/ Breathing Cycles	Continue cycles of 5 compressions and 1 breath. Recheck pulse every few minutes.		
Decision Making	Based on the information the instructor gives, make a decision about what to do next, and continue giving the appropriate care.		

Final Instructor Check _____

Skill Checklist: Airway Obstruction (Conscious Adult)

Remember: When practicing abdominal thrusts on a partner, do not give actual thrusts.

Critical Skill	Steps	PC	IC
Determine If Patient Is Choking	Determine if patient can cough, speak, or breathe. Ask, "Are you choking?"		
Shout for Help	Shout for help to attract another person's attention.		
Phone the EMS System for Help	Tell someone to call for an ambulance.		
Perform Abdominal Thrusts	Stand behind patient and wrap arms around patient's waist. Place thumb side of one fist against middle of patient's abdomen just above the navel and well below the lower tip of the breastbone. Grasp fist with your other hand and press into patient's abdomen with a quick upward thrust. Repeat thrusts until obstruction is cleared or patient becomes unconscious.		
Decision Making	Based on the information the instructor gives, make a decision about what to do next, and continue giving the appropriate care.		

Final Instructor Check _____

Skill Checklist: Airway Obstruction (Conscious Child)

Note: This checklist is included for your information only. You will not be tested on this skill.

Critical Skill	Steps
Determine If Child Is Choking	Determine if child can cough, speak, or breathe. Ask, "Are you choking?"
Shout for Help	Shout for help to attract another person's attention.
Phone the EMS System for Help	Tell someone to call for an ambulance.
Perform Abdominal Thrusts	Stand or kneel behind child and wrap arms around child's waist. Place thumb side of one fist against middle of child's abdomen just above the navel and well below the lower tip of the breastbone. Grasp fist with your other hand and press into child's abdomen with a quick upward thrust. Repeat thrusts until obstruction is cleared or child becomes unconscious.

Review and Fundamental Skills Checklists

Skill Checklist: Airway Obstruction (Conscious Infant)

Critical Skill	Steps	PC	IC
Determine If Infant Is Choking	Determine if infant can cry, cough, or breathe.		
Shout for Help	Shout for help to attract another person's attention.		
Phone the EMS System for Help	Tell someone to call for an ambulance.		
Give 4 Back Blows	Place infant face down along your forearm, with the head lower than the chest. Support the infant's head and neck by firmly holding the jaw. Rest forearm on your thigh. Give 4 back blows forcefully between the infant's shoulder blades.		
Locate Position for Chest Thrusts	Turn infant as a unit onto his or her back. Rest arm supporting infant on your thigh. Keep infant's head lower than the chest. Place pad of ring finger on infant's breastbone just below imaginary line connecting the nipples. Place pads of middle and index fingers next to ring finger, then raise ring finger. Pads of fingers should run down the length of the breastbone. If you feel the notch at the end of the infant's breastbone, move your fingers up the breastbone slightly.		
Give 4 Chest Thrusts	Compress breastbone 4 times, ½ to 1 inch, at a slower rate than chest compressions done during infant CPR.		
Repeat Back Blows and Chest Thrusts	Continue giving back blows and chest thrusts until obstruction is cleared or infant becomes unconscious.		
Decision Making	Based on the information the instructor gives, make a decision about what to do next, and continue giving the appropriate care.		

Final Instructor Check _____

Skill Checklist: Airway Obstruction (Unconscious Adult)

Remember: Do not perform finger sweeps on a manikin. Do not touch the manikin's lips or inside its mouth with your finger.

Critical Skill	Steps	PC	IC
Check for Unresponsiveness	Tap or gently shake patient. Shout, "Are you OK?"		
Shout for Help	Shout for help to attract another person's attention.		
Position the Patient	Roll patient onto back if necessary: place one hand on patient's shoulder and other hand on patient's hip and roll patient toward you as a unit. As you roll patient, support back of head and neck.		
Open the Airway	Using the head-tilt/chin-lift method, tilt head and lift jaw.		
Check for Breathlessness	Maintain open airway. Look at chest; listen and feel for breathing for 3 to 5 seconds.		
Give 2 Full Breaths	Maintain open airway. Pinch nose shut. Give 2 full breaths at the rate of 1 to 1½ seconds per breath.		
Retilt Patient's Head and Give 2 Full Breaths	If your breaths were unsuccessful, retilt patient's head. Maintain open airway. Pinch nose shut. Give 2 breaths at the rate of 1 to 1½ seconds per breath.		
Phone the EMS System for Help	Tell someone to call for an ambulance.		
Perform 6 to 10 Abdominal Thrusts	Straddle patient's thighs. Place heel of one hand against the middle of patient's abdomen just above the navel and well below the lower tip of breastbone. Place other hand directly on top of first hand. Press into patient's abdomen 6 to 10 times with quick upward thrusts.		
Do Finger Sweep (simulate)	Kneel beside patient's head. Open patient's mouth and grasp both tongue and lower jaw between thumb and fingers of hand nearest patient's legs; lift jaw. Insert index finger into patient's mouth along the inside of cheek and deep into throat to base of tongue. Dislodge and remove any foreign objects found.		
Give 2 Full Breaths	Maintain open airway. Pinch nose shut. Give 2 full breaths at the rate of 1 to 1½ seconds per breath.		
Repeat Sequence	Do 6 to 10 abdominal thrusts. Do finger sweep. Attempt to give 2 full breaths.		
Decision Making	Based on the information the instructor gives, make a decision about what to do next, and continue giving the appropriate care.		

Final Instructor Check _____

Review and Fundamental Skills Checklists

Skill Checklist: Airway Obstruction (Unconscious Child)

Note: This checklist is included for your information only. You will not be tested on this skill.

Critical Skill	Steps
Check for Unresponsiveness	Tap or gently shake child's shoulder. Shout, "Are you OK?"
Shout for Help	Shout for help to attract another person's attention.
Position the Child	Roll child onto back if necessary: place one hand on child's shoulder and other hand on child's hip, and roll child toward you as a unit. As you roll child, support back of head and neck.
Open the Airway	Using the head-tilt/chin-lift method, tilt the head gently back into the neutral-plus position; lift chin.
Check for Breathlessness	Maintain open airway. Look at chest and abdomen; listen and feel for breathing for 3 to 5 seconds.
Give 2 Slow Breaths	Maintain open airway. Pinch nose shut. Give 2 slow breaths at the rate of 1 to 1½ seconds per breath.
Retilt Child's Head and Give 2 Slow Breaths	If your breaths were unsuccessful, retilt child's head. Maintain open airway. Pinch nose shut. Give 2 slow breaths at the rate of 1 to 1½ seconds per breath.
Phone the EMS System for Help	Tell someone to call for an ambulance.
Perform 6 to 10 Abdominal Thrusts	Kneel at child's feet. (Straddle the thighs of a larger child if necessary.) Place heel of one hand against the middle of child's abdomen just above the navel and well below the lower tip of the breastbone. Place other hand directly on top of the first. Press into child's abdomen 6 to 10 times with quick upward thrusts.
Foreign Body Check (simulate)	Kneel beside child's head. Open child's mouth and grasp both tongue and lower jaw between thumb and fingers of hand nearest child's legs; lift jaw. Look inside mouth for object; if object is visible, attempt to remove it.
Give 2 Slow Breaths	Maintain open airway. Pinch nose shut. Give 2 slow breaths at the rate of 1 to 1½ seconds per breath.
Repeat Sequence	Do 6 to 10 abdominal thrusts. Do foreign body check. Attempt to give 2 slow breaths.

Skill Checklist: Airway Obstruction (Unconscious Infant)

Remember: Do not perform finger sweeps on a manikin. Do not touch the manikin's lips or inside its mouth with your finger.

Critical Skill	Steps	PC	IC
Check for Unresponsiveness	Tap or gently shake infant's shoulder.		
Shout for Help	Shout for help to attract another person's attention.		
Position the Infant	Roll infant onto back if necessary, supporting back of head and neck.		
Open the Airway	Using the head-tilt/chin-lift method, tilt the head gently back into the neutral position; lift chin.		
Check for Breathlessness	Maintain open airway. Look at chest and abdomen; listen and feel for breathing for 3 to 5 seconds.		
Give 2 Slow Breaths	Give 2 slow breaths at the rate of 1 to 1½ seconds per breath. Breathe into infant's mouth and nose.		
Retilt Infant's Head and Give 2 Slow Breaths	If your breaths were unsuccessful, retilt infant's head. Maintain open airway. Give 2 slow breaths at the rate of 1 to 1½ seconds per breath.		
Phone the EMS System for Help	Tell someone to call for an ambulance.		
Give 4 Back Blows	Place infant face down along your forearm, with the head lower than the chest. Support the infant's head and neck by firmly holding the jaw. Rest forearm on thigh. Give 4 back blows forcefully between the infant's shoulder blades.		
Locate Position for Chest Thrusts	Turn infant as a unit onto his or her back. Rest arm supporting infant on thigh. Keep infant's head lower than chest. Place pad of ring finger on infant's breastbone just below imaginary line connecting the nipples. Place pads of middle and index fingers next to ring finger, then raise ring finger. Pads of fingers should run down breastbone. If you feel the notch at the end of the infant's breastbone, move your fingers up the breastbone slightly.		
Give 4 Chest Thrusts	Compress breastbone 4 times, ½ to 1 inch, at a slower rate than chest compressions done during infant CPR.		
Foreign Body Check (simulate)	Open the mouth and grasp both tongue and lower jaw between thumb and fingers of hand nearest infant's legs; lift jaw. Look inside mouth for object; if object is seen, remove it.		
Give 2 Slow Breaths	Give 2 slow breaths at the rate of 1 to 1½ seconds per breath.		
Repeat Sequence	Give 4 back blows and 4 chest thrusts. Do foreign body check. Attempt to give 2 slow breaths.		
Decision Making	Based on the information the instructor gives, make a decision about what to do next, and continue giving the appropriate care.		

Final Instructor Check _____

Part II:
The Professional Rescuer Skills

Introduction to Part II

The professional rescuer skills taught and practiced in this course include the use of two-rescuer CPR for adults and children and the introduction of new methods to open the airway, in addition to the head-tilt/chin-lift. Participants will learn how to use the modified jaw thrust maneuver to open the airway in patients with suspected head, neck, or back injuries, how to give mouth-to-nose breathing, how to perform the triple airway maneuver, and how to use a resuscitation mask.

Directions for the Participant: Learning Professional Rescuer Skills

To complete the procedure for learning the skills in Part II of the professional rescuer course, the participants should do the following:

1. **Read** the narrative portion of the workbook that describes how the skill and its parts are performed.

2. **Complete** the review sections of the workbook.

3. **View** the video demonstration of the skill.

4. Using the skill sheets, **practice** the skill with a partner:
   a. One partner reads the steps aloud, while the other partner performs the step.
   b. The observing partner corrects any practice errors by telling the practicing partner the *correct* changes needed. Direct statements of how the skill should be performed provide the partner who is practicing the skills with immediate clues for correction.

5. **Review** the video demonstration of the skill at any time by replaying the videocassette when needed. A quick look at how the skill is performed can save time and energy, as this provides the participant with the visual clues needed to continue making progress with minimal interruption.

6. Using the skill checklists, **request** a skill check—first from the partner and then from the instructor:
   a. The practicing partner requests a skill check from the observing partner when he or she feels able to perform the skills correctly without prompting. The observing partner checks off each step in the Partner Check (PC) column on the skill checklist.

b. One or both partners request(s) a final skill check from the instructor when ready to demonstrate the skill. The instructor checks off the skill in the Instructor Check (IC) column on the skill checklist. The participant must get the instructor's signature on the bottom of each skill checklist to document correct performance of the skills.

Participants needing more practice time are asked to continue practice in that skill before moving on to the next skill in the sequence.

Upon satisfactory completion of the professional rescuer skills, participants will take a written test.

Disease Transmission and Performance of CPR by the Professional Rescuer

Evidence shows that lay rescuers are far more likely to use rescue breathing and CPR on members of their own family than on strangers. As professional rescuers, however, participants in this course can expect to come into contact with a wider range of the population when providing emergency care. For this reason, additional information on disease transmission has been included.

The following guidelines, "Recommendations for Prevention of HIV Transmission in Health Care Settings," were established by the Centers for Disease Control (CDC) in 1987. Red Cross instructors for this course also receive periodic updates concerning disease transmission. Questions about the information included in this section and other questions about disease transmission should be directed to the instructor.

Recommendations for Prevention of HIV Transmission in Health Care Settings

These guidelines have been excerpted from *Morbidity and Mortality Weekly Report (MMWR) Supplement,* August 1987, Vol. 36, No. 2S., U.S. Department of Health and Human Services, Public Health Service, Centers for Disease Control, Atlanta.

Introduction

Human immunodeficiency virus (HIV), the virus that causes acquired immunodeficiency syndrome (AIDS), is transmitted through sexual contact and exposure to infected blood or blood components and perinatally from mother to neonate (newborn). HIV has been isolated from blood, semen, vaginal secretions, saliva, tears, breast milk, cerebrospinal fluid, and urine, and is likely to be isolated from other body fluids, secretions, and excretions. However, epidemiologic evidence has implicated only blood, semen, vaginal secretions, and possibly breast milk in transmission.

The increasing prevalence of HIV increases the risk that health-care workers will be exposed to blood from patients infected with HIV, especially when blood and body-fluid precautions are not followed for all patients. Thus, this document emphasizes the need for health-care workers to consider *all* patients as potentially infected with HIV and/or other blood-borne pathogens, and to adhere rigorously to infection-control precautions for minimizing the risk of exposure to blood and body fluids of all patients.

The recommendations contained in this document consolidate and update CDC recommendations published earlier for preventing HIV transmission in health-care settings: (1) precautions for clinical and laboratory staffs; (2) precautions for health-care workers and allied professionals; (3) recommendations for preventing HIV transmission in the workplace. . . . The recommendations . . . have been developed for use in health-care settings and emphasize the need to treat blood and other body fluids from *all* patients as potentially infective. These same prudent precautions also should be taken *in other settings* in which persons may be exposed to blood or other body fluids.

Definition of Health-Care Workers

Health-care workers are defined as persons, including students and trainees, whose activities involve contact with patients or with blood or other body fluids from patients in a health-care setting. . .

Precautions to Prevent Transmission of HIV

Universal Precautions

Since medical history and examination cannot reliably identify all patients infected with HIV or other blood-borne pathogens, blood and body-fluid precautions should be consistently used for *all* patients. This approach, previously recommended by CDC, and referred to as "universal blood and body-fluid precautions" or "universal precautions," should be used in the care of *all* patients, especially including those in emergency-care settings in which the risk of blood exposure is increased and the infection status of the patient is usually unknown[1].

1. All health-care workers should routinely use appropriate barrier precautions to prevent skin and mucous-membrane exposure when contact with blood or other body fluids of any patient is anticipated. Gloves should be worn for touching blood and body fluids, mucous membranes, or non-intact skin of all patients, for handling items or surfaces soiled with blood or body fluids, and for performing venipuncture and other vascular access procedures. Gloves should be changed after contact with each patient. Masks and protective eyewear or face shields should be worn during procedures that are likely to generate droplets of blood or other body fluids to prevent exposure of mucous membranes of the mouth, nose, and eyes. Gowns or aprons should be worn during procedures that are likely to generate splashes of blood or other body fluids.

2. Hands and other skin surfaces should be washed immediately and thoroughly if contaminated with blood or other body fluids. Hands should be washed immediately after gloves are removed.

3. All health-care workers should take precautions to prevent injuries caused by needles, scalpels, and other sharp instruments or devices during procedures; when cleaning used instruments; during disposal of used needles; and when handling sharp instruments after procedures. To prevent needlestick injuries, needles should not be recapped, purposely bent or broken by hand, removed from disposable syringes, or otherwise manipulated by hand. After they are used, disposable syringes and needles, scalpel blades, and other sharp items should be placed in puncture-resistant containers for disposal; the puncture-resistant containers should be located as close as practical to the use area. Large-bore reusable needles should be placed in a puncture-resistant container for transport to the reprocessing area.

4. Although saliva has not been implicated in HIV transmission, to minimize the need for emergency mouth-to-mouth resuscitation, mouthpieces, resuscitation bags, or other ventilation devices should be available for use in areas in which the need for resuscitation is predictable.

5. Health-care workers who have exudative lesions or weeping dermatitis should refrain from all direct patient care and from handling patient-care equipment until the condition resolves.

6. Pregnant health-care workers are not known to be at greater risk of contracting HIV infection than health-care workers who are not pregnant; however, if a health-care worker develops HIV infection during pregnancy, the infant is at risk of infection resulting from perinatal transmission. Because of this risk, pregnant health-care workers should be especially familiar with and strictly adhere to precautions to minimize the risk of HIV transmission. . . .

[1]Baker, J.L., G.D. Kelen, K.T. Sivertson, T.C. Quinn. 1987. "Unsuspected human immunodeficiency virus in critically ill emergency patients." *JAMA* 257: 2609–11.

•6 *Two-rescuer CPR*

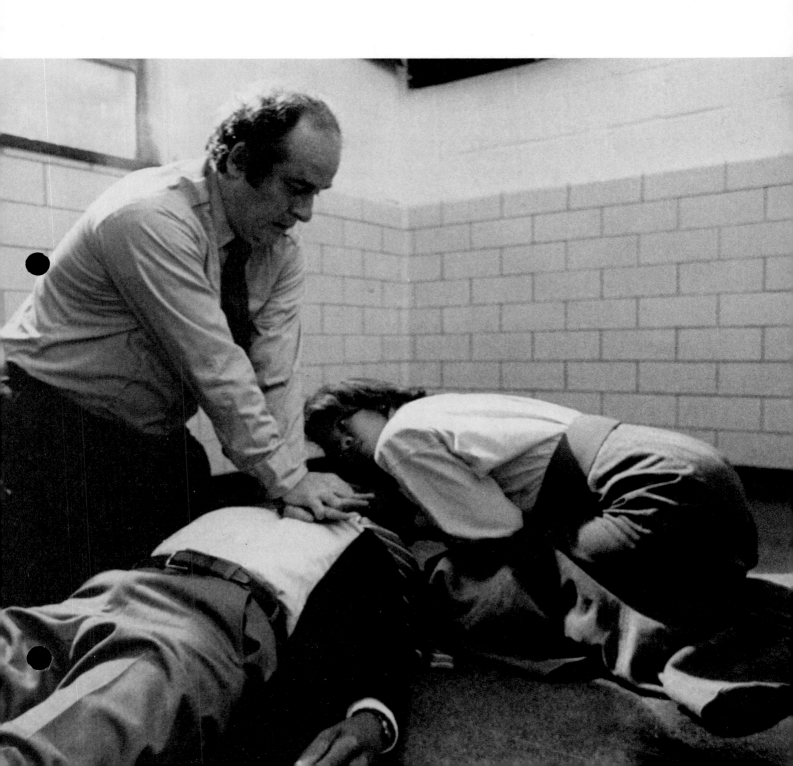

MAIN IDEAS

1. Two-rescuer CPR is a skill primarily taught to professional rescuers and performed on adults and on children aged approximately one through eight.
2. Two-rescuer CPR is started (1) when CPR is already in progress and a second rescuer arrives to assist, and (2) when two professional rescuers arrive at the scene of an emergency at the same time.
3. It is important for professional rescuers to know how and when to change positions during two-rescuer CPR.

CHAPTER OUTLINE

I. Performing Two-rescuer Adult CPR
II. Performing Two-rescuer Child CPR
III. Review
IV. Practice Sessions
   A. Two professional rescuers starting CPR together
   B. Two-rescuer CPR—changing positions
   C. Addition of a second rescuer when one rescuer is already performing CPR

OBJECTIVES

1. Describe and demonstrate two-rescuer CPR under various conditions.
2. Describe the specific procedures used in two-rescuer CPR for adults and for children.

Performing Two-rescuer Adult CPR

Two-rescuer CPR is a procedure in which two people share the responsibility for performing rescue breathing and chest compressions. These skills build on but are different from the single-rescuer skills taught in other American Red Cross CPR courses. How and when the professional rescuer begins two-rescuer CPR depends on several factors. In many cases, the second rescuer enters after one-rescuer CPR has already been started. The professional rescuer can begin or take over CPR in the following situations:

1. CPR is *not* in progress and two or more professional rescuers arrive on the scene at the same time and begin two-rescuer CPR together.

2. One-rescuer CPR is in progress by a professional rescuer and a second rescuer is available to begin two-rescuer CPR.

3. One-rescuer CPR is in progress and the rescuer is tired and needs to be relieved. (In this case, one-person CPR is taken over by the second rescuer.)

Two-rescuer Techniques and Procedures

Whenever two-rescuer adult CPR is performed, there are standard techniques and procedures to follow. During two-rescuer adult CPR:

- Five compressions are given followed by 1 breath (a ratio of 5 to 1).

- Chest compressions are given at the rate of 80 to 100 per minute, and at a depth of 1½ to 2 inches (3.8 to 5 cm) (the same as in one-rescuer CPR).

- The compressor (rescuer giving compressions) uses the same counting rhythm as for one-rescuer CPR: "One-and, two-and, three-and, four-and, five;"–(breath)–"One-and, two-and, three-and, four-and, five."

- Compressions are stopped at the upstroke of the fifth compression, and the ventilator (rescuer giving ventilations) immediately gives 1 full breath for 1 to 1½ seconds. The compressor then continues with compressions.

- The ventilator monitors the effectiveness of the compressions by checking the carotid pulse while the compressor is compressing. He or she informs the compressor whether or not the compressions are effective. Note that sometimes, if the patient has lost a significant amount of blood, there will not be enough blood volume to register a carotid pulse, even though compressions are effective.

• The ventilator does a pulse check after the first minute of compressions and every few minutes after that in order to determine if spontaneous circulation has returned. He or she says, "Pulse check," and the compressor stops compressing after the fifth compression. The ventilator checks the pulse for 5 seconds, says, "Has pulse" or "No pulse," and gives 1 breath. The rescuers continue performing two-rescuer CPR.

• During two-rescuer CPR, if the rescuers need to change positions, there is a set procedure to follow (see page 69).

When Two Professional Rescuers Arrive on the Scene at the Same Time

When two professional rescuers arrive on the scene at the same time, they have usually been sent by an EMS system. If CPR is not being performed, one rescuer goes to the patient, does a primary survey and, if appropriate, begins CPR. The other handles responsibilities at the scene such as radio communications, equipment and supply setup, and calming the patient's family or friends.

Two Rescuers Beginning CPR Together

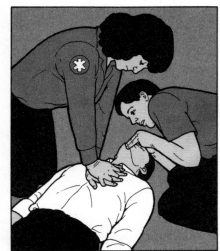

Figure 15
Two-rescuer CPR

In situations where both rescuers are available to begin CPR at the same time, the *first* rescuer:

1. Checks for unresponsiveness.
2. Shouts for help.
3. Positions the patient.
4. Gets into position at the patient's head.
5. Opens the airway.
6. Checks for breathlessness.
7. Says, "No breathing" if no breathing.
8. Gives 2 full breaths.
9. Checks for pulse.
10. Says, "No pulse, begin CPR."

While the first rescuer is completing the primary survey, the *second* rescuer:

1. Locates the landmark for chest compressions.
2. Assumes the correct hand position.
3. Begins chest compressions after first rescuer says, "No pulse, begin CPR."

Both rescuers continue CPR together *(Fig. 15).*

Two-rescuer CPR: Changing Positions

When the rescuer doing compressions gets tired, both rescuers change positions. Even though either rescuer may become tired, the call to switch positions is made by the compressor. When the switch is made, the rescuer at the patient's head completes one breath and then moves immediately to the chest and becomes the compressor; the rescuer at the chest moves immediately to the head and becomes the ventilator. Both rescuers move quickly into position without changing sides *(Fig. 16)*. The sequence for changing positions is the following:

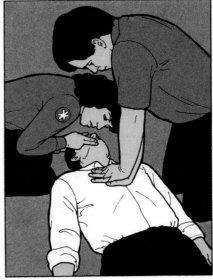

Figure 16
Two-rescuer CPR After Changing Positions

1. The compressor tells the ventilator in advance that he or she wants to change positions at the end of the next cycle.

2. The compressor begins the cycle of compressions by saying, "*Change*-and two-and three-and four-and five."

3. The ventilator gives 1 breath to complete the cycle after the fifth compression.

4. After giving the breath, the rescuer at the head moves to the chest and becomes the compressor. He or she gets into position, locates the landmark, and positions his or her hands for compressions.

5. After giving the last compression, the rescuer at the chest moves to the head and becomes the ventilator. He or she checks the carotid pulse for 5 seconds and, if there is no pulse, says, "No pulse, continue CPR" and gives 1 breath.

6. The rescuers continue performing two-rescuer CPR.

When CPR Is in Progress By One Rescuer

When one-rescuer CPR is in progress and a second rescuer comes to the scene, that rescuer should ask whether the EMS system has been called. If not, he or she calls the EMS system. Then the second rescuer either *replaces* the first rescuer, or *assists* him or her in giving two-rescuer CPR.

When arriving on the scene, the *second* rescuer:

1. Identifies him or herself as a professional rescuer; says, "I know CPR. Can I help?"
2. If the rescuer has not been sent by EMS, he or she asks, "Have you called EMS?"
3. Calls the EMS system if necessary.
4. Either takes over one-rescuer CPR or joins the first rescuer in giving two-rescuer CPR.

Two Professional Rescuers Taking Over CPR From One Rescuer Performing CPR

When two professional rescuers arrive at the scene at the same time and one-rescuer CPR *is* in progress, they may take over from the person performing CPR. The two-person team begins immediately after a cycle of 15 compressions and 2 breaths is completed. In that case, the *first* rescuer:

1. Gets into position at the patient's head.
2. Opens the airway.
3. Checks the carotid pulse.
4. If no pulse, says, "No pulse, continue CPR."
5. Gives 1 breath.

The *second* rescuer:

1. Gets into position at the patient's chest.
2. Locates the proper hand position.
3. Begins chest compressions after the partner gives 1 breath.

Addition of a Second Rescuer When One Rescuer Is Already Performing CPR

If one professional rescuer is already performing CPR, and a second professional rescuer becomes available *(Fig. 17)*, two-rescuer CPR is begun as follows:

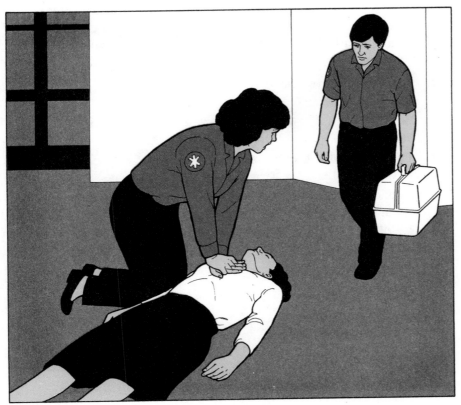

Figure 17
Arrival of a Second Rescuer

The second rescuer enters immediately after the first rescuer has completed a full cycle of 15 compressions and 2 breaths.

The *second* rescuer:

1. Gets into position at the patient's chest.
2. Locates the landmark and assumes the correct hand position.

The *first* rescuer:

1. Remains at the patient's head.
2. Checks the carotid pulse.
3. If no pulse says, "No pulse, continue CPR."
4. Gives 1 breath.

The *second* rescuer, at the chest, begins chest compressions. They continue giving two-rescuer CPR.

Performing Two-rescuer Child CPR

Two-rescuer CPR can also be performed on children (aged approximately one through eight). With large children, it is sometimes necessary to use adult CPR techniques.

Most of the procedures for two-rescuer child CPR are similar to those used in two-rescuer adult CPR. The same ratio of compressions to ventilations is used for children as for adults. The procedures for assessing the patient's condition and changing places are also the same. However, there are four major differences:

1. In child CPR, the head is tilted gently back into the neutral-plus position.

2. In child CPR, chest compressions are performed with one hand only.

3. The depth of the compressions is shallower for children: 1 to 1½ inches (2.5 to 3.8 cm).

4. Depending on the size of the child, a smaller volume of air is given to a child than to an adult in rescue breathing. The amount of air should be just enough to make the chest rise.

Review

Indicate whether each of the following statements about performing two-rescuer CPR is true or false by checking "True" or "False."

Statement	TRUE	FALSE
1. One breath is given after every 5 compressions.	☐	☐
2. The rescuer at the head checks the pulse.	☐	☐
3. The compressor stops after the fifth compression for 4 to 5 seconds while the ventilator gives 1 full breath.	☐	☐
4. The rescuer at the chest begins compressions after the rescuer at the head says, "No pulse."	☐	☐
5. Compressions in two-rescuer CPR are given at a different rate than they are in one-rescuer CPR.	☐	☐
6. In order to determine the effectiveness of compressions, the ventilator checks the pulse while the chest is being compressed.	☐	☐
7. When one rescuer wants to change positions, the call to change positions is made by the ventilator.	☐	☐
8. When two rescuers change positions, the rescuer at the head completes 1 breath after the fifth compression and then moves to the chest.	☐	☐
9. When two rescuers change positions, the first thing the rescuer does after moving to the head is give 1 breath.	☐	☐
10. CPR for children is done exactly the same as CPR for adults.	☐	☐

Answers

1. **True.** One breath is given after every 5 compressions.

2. **True.** The rescuer at the head checks the pulse.

3. **False.** The pause time between compressions for the breath is *1 to 1½ seconds.*

4. **True.** The rescuer at the chest begins compressions after the rescuer at the head says, "No pulse."

5. **False.** Compressions in two-rescuer CPR are given at *the same rate* as for one-rescuer CPR: *80 to 100 compressions per minute.*

6. **True.** In order to determine the effectiveness of compressions, the ventilator checks the pulse while the chest is being compressed.

7. **False.** When one rescuer gets tired, the call to change positions is made by the *compressor.*

8. **True.** When two rescuers change positions, the rescuer at the head completes 1 breath after the fifth compression and then moves to the chest.

9. **False.** The first thing the rescuer at the chest does after moving to the head is *check the carotid pulse for 5 seconds.*

10. **False.** There are *four major differences* between adult CPR and child CPR. In child CPR:
    a. The head is tilted gently back into the neutral-plus position.
    b. Chest compressions are performed with one hand only.
    c. The depth of the compressions is shallower for children (from 1 to 1½ inches) (2.5 to 3.8 cm).
    d. A smaller volume of air is given to a child (just enough to make the chest rise).

Practice Session: Two-rescuer CPR

During the practice for two-rescuer CPR, there is no opportunity to decontaminate the manikin when participants practice changing positions. In order to limit the potential for disease transmission during this exercise, *the second participant taking over the ventilation should simulate ventilation instead of blowing into the manikin.*

Note: The use of the resuscitation mask in two-rescuer CPR is taught in Chapter 8 (see skill sheet, page 111).

Practice Session: Two Professional Rescuers Beginning CPR Together

You and another professional rescuer arrive on the scene at the same time. After completing the primary survey and, if necessary, sending another person to call the EMS system, you and your partner begin two-rescuer CPR.

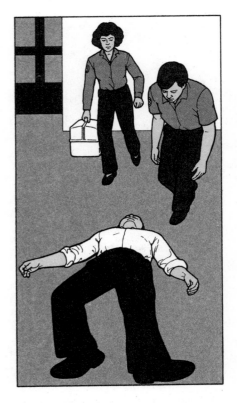

PRIMARY SURVEY

AIRWAY

BREATHING

CIRCULATION

Skill Sheet:

First Rescuer (Ventilator)

Check for unresponsiveness.

Shout for help.

Position the patient.

Take position at patient's head.

Open the airway.

Check for breathlessness.

Say, "No breathing."

Give 2 full breaths.

Feel for carotid pulse for 5 to 10 seconds.

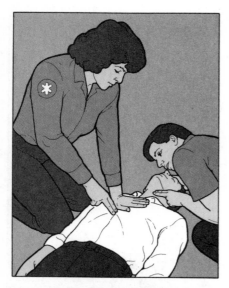

Second Rescuer (Compressor)

Kneel at patient's chest.

Locate landmark for chest compressions while first rescuer begins to check for pulse.

Assume correct hand position.

First Rescuer (Ventilator)

Say, "No pulse, begin CPR."

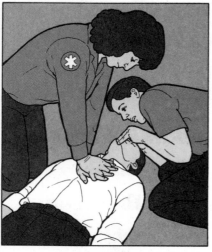

Second Rescuer (Compressor)

Start chest compressions at a ratio of 5 compressions to 1 breath.

Count out loud, "One-and, two-and, three-and, four-and, five."

Stop compressions after each cycle of 5 and allow first rescuer to give 1 breath.

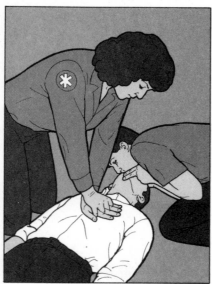

First Rescuer (Ventilator)

After every fifth compression, give 1 full breath, lasting 1 to 1½ seconds.

Check compression effectiveness by checking pulse while your partner is giving compressions.

At the end of the first minute, say, "Pulse check" and feel for carotid pulse for 5 seconds.

Say, "No pulse, continue CPR."

Give 1 breath.

Recheck pulse every few minutes as you continue two-rescuer CPR.

Practice Session: Two-rescuer CPR— Changing Positions

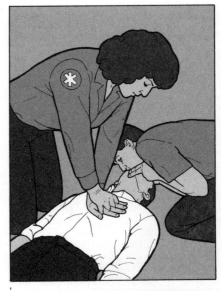

You and another professional rescuer arrive on the scene at the same time. After completing the primary survey and, if necessary, sending another person to call the EMS system, you and your partner begin two-rescuer CPR.

When the rescuer giving compressions gets tired, the rescuers change positions. Even though either rescuer may get tired, the call to switch is made by the compressor.

After completing several cycles of CPR, the rescuers change places.

Skill Sheet:

Compressor

Say, "*Change*-and, two-and, three-and, four-and, five."

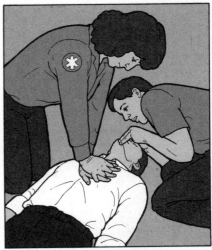

Ventilator

Complete 1 breath as usual at end of "*change*" cycle.

Move quickly to patient's chest and become compressor.

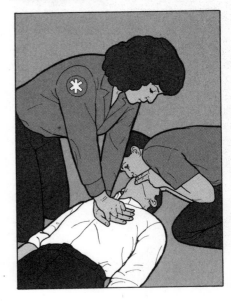

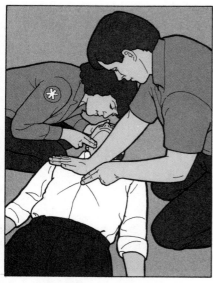

Compressor

Move quickly to patient's head and become ventilator.

New Ventilator

Feel for carotid pulse for 5 seconds.

New Compressor

Get into position, locate landmark, and position hands for compressions.

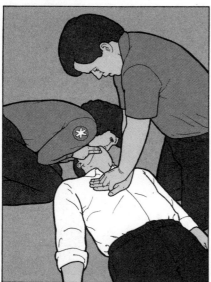

New Ventilator

Say, "No pulse, continue CPR."

Give 1 breath.

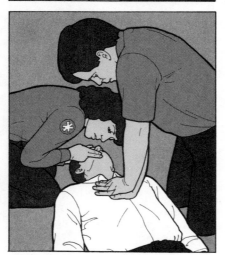

New Compressor

Begin compressions after ventilator checks pulse, says, "No pulse, continue CPR," and gives 1 breath.

Compress chest immediately after the breath is given, and continue the cycle.

Practice Session: Addition of a Second Rescuer When One Rescuer Is Already Performing CPR

If one professional rescuer is already performing CPR, and a second professional rescuer becomes available, two-rescuer CPR is begun as follows. This practice begins while the first rescuer is performing one-rescuer CPR.

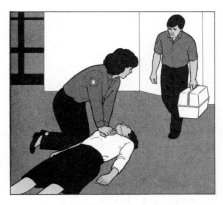

Skill Sheet:

Second Rescuer (Person Entering)

Identify yourself as a professional rescuer. Say, "I know CPR. Have you called EMS?"

Call the EMS system if first rescuer has not.

First Rescuer

Give 2 breaths, completing the cycle.

Second Rescuer (Compressor)

As first rescuer completes full cycle of 15 compressions and 2 breaths, get into position at patient's chest.

Locate landmark and assume correct hand position.

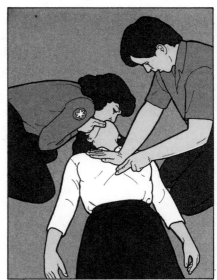

First Rescuer (Ventilator)

Say, "Pulse check" and feel for carotid pulse for 5 seconds.

If no pulse say, "No pulse, continue CPR."

Give 1 breath.

Second Rescuer (Compressor)

Start chest compressions at a ratio of 5 compressions to 1 breath.

Skill Checklist: Two Professional Rescuers
Beginning CPR Together

Critical Skill	Steps	PC	IC
First Rescuer (Ventilator) Do a Primary Survey	Check for unresponsiveness. Shout for help. Position the patient. Open the airway. Check for breathlessness. Give 2 full breaths. Feel for carotid pulse for 5 to 10 seconds.		
Second Rescuer (Compressor) Locate Compression Position Give 5 Compressions	Locate landmark for chest compressions while ventilator checks for pulse. Assume correct hand position. After ventilator says, "No pulse, begin CPR," give 5 compressions. Stop after the fifth compression and allow ventilator to give 1 breath.		
Ventilator Give 1 Full Breath	After fifth compression, give 1 full breath.		
Do Compression/ Breathing Cycles	Do 12 cycles of 5 compressions and 1 breath. Ventilator monitors effectiveness of compressions by checking pulse while partner is compressing.		
Ventilator Recheck Pulse	At end of first minute, say, "Pulse check," and feel for carotid pulse for 5 seconds.		
Decision Making	Based on the information the instructor gives, make a decision about what to do next, and continue giving the appropriate care.		

Final Instructor Check _____

Skill Checklist: Two-rescuer CPR— Changing Positions

Note: The second rescuer taking over the ventilation should simulate ventilation instead of blowing into the manikin.

Critical Skill	Steps	PC	IC
Do Compression/ Breathing Cycles	Do 12 cycles of 5 compressions and 1 breath.		
Compressor Signal Change	Say, "*Change*-and, two-and, three-and, four-and, five."		
Ventilator Give 1 Full Breath	At the end of the change cycle, give 1 full breath.		
Rescuers Change Positions	Compressor moves to patient's head and becomes new ventilator. Ventilator moves to patient's chest and becomes new compressor.		
New Ventilator Check Pulse	Feel for carotid pulse for 5 seconds.		
New Compressor Locate Compression Position	Locate landmark and position hands for compressions while new ventilator checks for pulse.		
New Ventilator Give 1 Full Breath	Say, "No pulse, continue CPR." Give 1 full breath.		
New Compressor Give 5 Compressions	Give 5 compressions. Pause after fifth compression to allow ventilator to give 1 breath.		
Decision Making	Based on the information the instructor gives, make a decision about what to do next, and continue giving the appropriate care.		

Final Instructor Check _____

Skill Checklist: Addition of a Second Rescuer When One Rescuer Is Already Performing CPR

Critical Skill	Steps	PC	IC
Second Rescuer Identify Yourself and Phone the EMS System for Help	Identify yourself as a professional rescuer. Phone the EMS system if the first rescuer has not.		
First Rescuer Give 2 Full Breaths	Give 2 full breaths completing the one-rescuer cycle of 15 compressions and 2 breaths.		
Second Rescuer (Compressor) Locate Compression Position	Get into position at patient's chest. Locate landmark and assume correct hand position.		
First Rescuer (Ventilator) Check Pulse and Give 1 Full Breath	Feel for carotid pulse for 5 seconds. If no pulse, say, "No pulse, continue CPR." Give 1 full breath.		
Compressor Give Chest Compressions	Give chest compressions at a ratio of 5 compressions to 1 breath.		
Decision Making	Based on the information the instructor gives, make a decision about what to do next, and continue giving the appropriate care.		

Final Instructor Check _____

●7 *Airway Management*

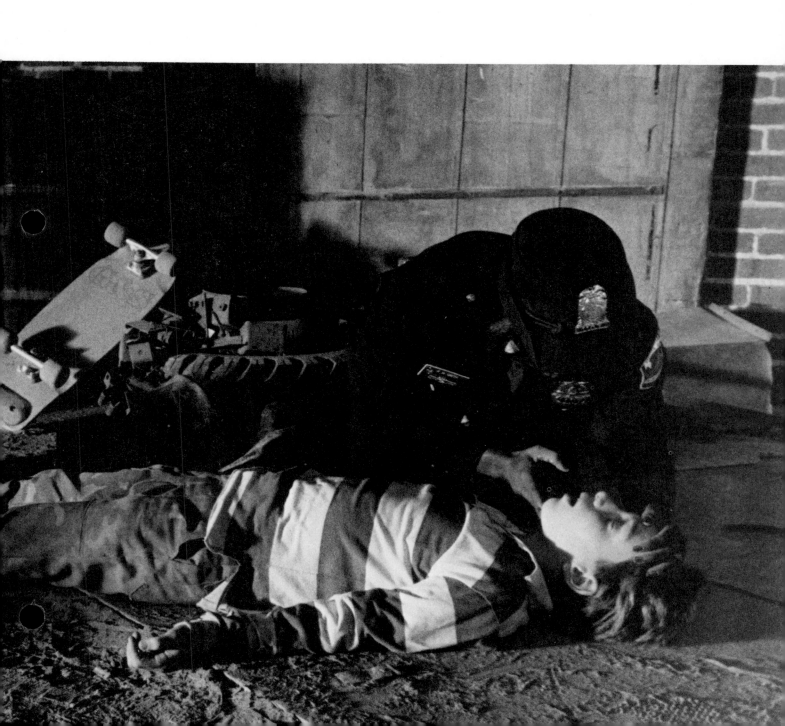

MAIN IDEAS

1. Knowing how to open a patient's airway and give rescue breathing under emergency conditions is a critical skill.
2. Professional rescuers should know alternative methods of opening the airway: the triple airway maneuver and the modified jaw thrust.
3. The triple airway maneuver is used to open a patient's airway when using a resuscitation mask, and the modified jaw thrust is used when a head, neck, or back injury is suspected.
4. Professional rescuers also need to know how to deliver mouth-to-nose rescue breathing and mouth-to-stoma rescue breathing.
5. Breathing too much air into a patient can cause gastric distention and vomiting.

CHAPTER OUTLINE

I. Importance of Airway Management
II. Two Additional Methods of Opening the Airway
   A. Triple airway maneuver
   B. Modified jaw thrust
III. Other Rescue Breathing Techniques
   A. Mouth-to-nose
   B. Mouth-to-stoma
IV. Gastric Distention
V. Review
VI. Practice Sessions
   A. Modified jaw thrust
   B. Mouth-to-nose rescue breathing

OBJECTIVES

1. Describe when the triple airway maneuver and the modified jaw thrust are used.
2. Describe how the professional rescuer performs mouth-to-nose and mouth-to-stoma rescue breathing.
3. Identify two consequences of breathing too much air into a patient.
4. Demonstrate the modified jaw thrust and mouth-to-nose rescue breathing.

Background: The Importance of Airway Management

The professional rescuer is called upon to assist victims in many different kinds of emergencies. A common life-threatening situation involves people who have stopped breathing. When the primary survey shows that a person has stopped breathing, rescue breathing must begin without delay. The most important action for successful resuscitation is the immediate opening of the airway. Basic CPR courses teach the lay rescuer the head-tilt/chin-lift method of opening a victim's airway. The head-tilt/chin-lift is the easiest way to open the airway, and can be used when the rescuer does not suspect a head, neck, or back injury.

This course presents two additional methods of opening the airway: the **triple airway maneuver** and the **modified jaw thrust.** The triple airway maneuver can be more effective (although more difficult to do) than the head-tilt/chin-lift, and it is the recommended technique for opening the airway when the rescuer uses a resuscitation mask. The modified jaw thrust minimizes head and neck movement, and it is used *when a head, neck, or back injury is suspected.*

The Triple Airway Maneuver

The triple airway maneuver is considered the most effective way to open the airway of a patient who does not have a spinal injury. It can be used to open the airway when other techniques are ineffective, and it is used in the application of a resuscitation mask when the patient does not have a spinal injury. (The procedure is taught in Chapter 8.)

As the name suggests, the triple airway maneuver has three parts. The rescuer: (1) tilts the patient's head back; (2) lifts the jaw upward; and (3) opens the patient's mouth. Done in sequence, these three steps open the airway *(Fig. 18).*

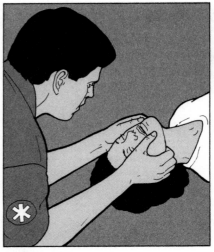

Figure 18
Triple Airway Maneuver

The Modified Jaw Thrust Maneuver for Adults, Children, and Infants

The modified jaw thrust maneuver is used to open the airway when the rescuer suspects that the patient has a head, neck, or back injury, because it minimizes head and neck movement.

A head, neck, or back (spinal cord) injury should always be suspected in patients who have been in a violent accident or who have suffered a traumatic injury, particularly if the trauma might have subjected the spine to sudden acceleration or deceleration.

This could be from an automobile accident, fall, diving accident, or other sports-related accident *(Fig. 19)*. If there is a head injury and the patient is unconscious, the rescuer should suspect a spinal cord injury.

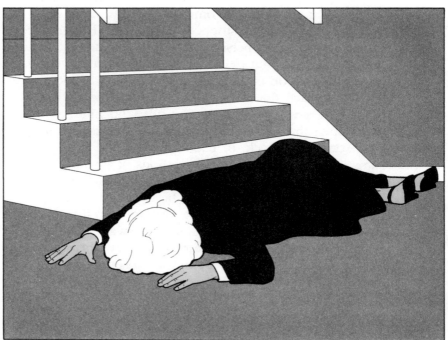

Figure 19
Possible Head, Neck, or Back Injury From a Fall

If a spinal cord injury is suspected, the rescuer immediately kneels behind the patient and stabilizes the patient's head and neck (keeps the head still). The rescuer places his or her hands along both sides of the patient's head with the fingers touching the jaw line to prevent the head from moving from side to side or forward and backward. This technique is known as "in-line stabilization" because it keeps the head in line with the spine.

Then, during the primary survey, when checking for unresponsiveness in a patient who may have a head, neck, or back injury, the rescuer *asks,* rather than shouts, "Are you OK?" This is done so the patient is not startled, which might cause him or her to move or jerk in surprise, causing further injury.

If a head, neck, or back injury is suspected, the head should not be turned to the side or the body moved. If moving the patient is necessary to deliver basic life support, the head, neck, and back should be supported and turned as a unit. It is recommended that more than one person help turn the patient, working together so the patient is rolled over as one unit. The modified jaw thrust maneuver should then be used to open the airway.

To perform the modified jaw thrust, the rescuer kneels at an angle behind the patient's head, positions his or her elbows on the surface on which the patient is lying, and rests his or her hands on both sides of the patient's head to support it and keep it immobile. The rescuer places the fingers of both hands under the patient's lower jaw just in front of the earlobes, positions the thumbs across the patient's cheekbones, and then applies pressure upward to lift the jaw forward and open the airway *(Fig. 20)*. The rescuer then performs rescue breathing, following the steps in the skill sheet on page 92.

The skill sheet for the modified jaw thrust includes the following new skills:

- Checking for suspected head, neck, or back injury.
- Closing off the patient's nostrils with the rescuer's cheek during ventilation when a head, neck, or back injury is suspected.
- Checking the carotid pulse while maintaining in-line stabilization.

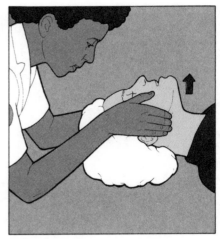

Figure 20
Modified Jaw Thrust

A skill sheet showing the techniques for using the modified jaw thrust with a resuscitation mask is included on page 109 in Chapter 8.

Mouth-to-Nose Rescue Breathing

There are a few situations when the rescuer may not be able to make a tight enough seal over a patient's mouth to perform mouth-to-mouth rescue breathing. For example, the patient's jaw or mouth may be injured during an accident, the jaw may be shut too tight to open, or the rescuer's mouth may be too small. In such cases, mouth-to-nose rescue breathing should be done as follows:

- The rescuer maintains the backward head-tilt position with one hand on the patient's forehead, and uses the other hand to close the mouth, being sure to push on the chin and not on the throat.

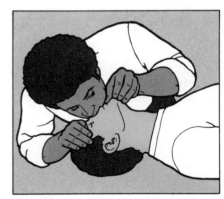

Figure 21
Mouth-to-Nose Breathing

- The rescuer opens his or her mouth wide, takes a deep breath, seals his or her mouth tightly around the patient's nose and breathes full breaths into the nose *(Fig. 21)*, doing the skill as described for the mouth-to-mouth method. The patient's mouth should be opened between breaths, if possible, to allow air to come out.

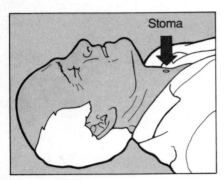

Figure 22
Patient With a Stoma

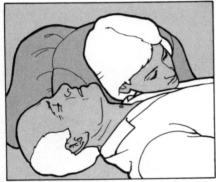

Figure 23
Check for Breathing

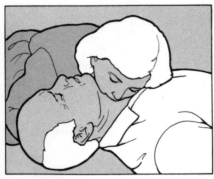

Figure 24
Mouth-to-Stoma Breathing

Mouth-to-Stoma Rescue Breathing

Some people have had surgery to remove all or part of the upper end of their windpipe. They breathe through an opening called a **stoma** in the front of the neck *(Fig. 22).* The stoma takes the air right into the windpipe, bypassing both the mouth and nose.

Most people with this condition wear a special bracelet or necklace or carry a card identifying their condition. In an emergency, the professional rescuer may not have time to search for a medical card, so it is important to look at the front of the neck during the primary survey to see if the person has a stoma.

Rescue breathing for someone with a stoma is given through the stoma—not through the mouth or nose.

In mouth-to-stoma rescue breathing, the rescuer uses the same basic steps as in mouth-to-mouth rescue breathing, except that the rescuer should—

1. Look, listen, and feel for breathing, with the ear held over the stoma *(Fig. 23).*

2. Give breaths into the stoma, breathing at the same rate as for mouth-to-mouth breathing *(Fig. 24).*

There are several other important things to remember when giving rescue breathing to someone who breathes through a stoma.

The rescuer—

• Should not tilt the patient's head back.

• Should not breathe air into the patient through the patient's nose or mouth. This may fill the patient's stomach with air.

• Should never block the stoma, which is the only way the patient has to breathe.

In some instances, a person who has had only part of the upper end of his or her windpipe removed may breathe through the stoma, as well as through the nose and mouth. If the patient's chest does not rise when the rescuer breathes through the stoma, he or she should close off the patient's mouth and nose *(Fig. 25)* and continue breathing through the stoma.

Gastric Distention (Air in the Stomach)

Sometimes during rescue breathing, air may enter the patient's stomach. Air in the stomach can be a serious problem, as it can make the patient vomit. When an unconscious person vomits, the stomach contents may be **aspirated** into the lungs, which may be fatal to the patient.

Air can enter the stomach three ways:

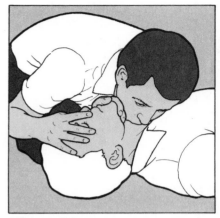

Figure 25
Mouth-to-Stoma Breathing for Partial Stoma

- When the rescuer keeps breathing into the patient after the chest has risen, causing extra air to fill the stomach.

- When the rescuer has not tilted the patient's head back far enough to open the airway completely, and must therefore breathe with greater pressure to fill the patient's lungs.

- When the rescue breaths are given too quickly. Quick breaths are given with higher pressure, causing air to enter the stomach.

To avoid forcing air into the stomach, the rescuer must be sure to keep the patient's head tilted far enough back. The rescuer should breathe into the patient only enough to make the chest rise. Breaths should not be given too quickly; the rescuer should pause between breaths long enough to let the patient's lungs empty and to take another breath.

If the rescuer notices that the patient's stomach has begun to bulge, he or she must make sure that the head is tilted back far enough and that he or she is not breathing into the patient too hard or too fast.

Vomiting

The unconscious patient may vomit while rescue breathing is being administered. If this happens, the rescuer should turn the patient's head and body to the side, quickly wipe the vomit out of the patient's mouth, and continue where he or she left off.

Review

Check the correct answer.

1. A rescuer should use the _____ to open the airway if he or she suspects that the patient has a head, neck, or back injury.
   - ☐ a. Head-tilt/chin-lift.
   - ☐ b. Modified jaw thrust.
   - ☐ c. Triple airway maneuver.
   - ☐ d. Chin-lift with head-tilt.

2. A _____ should always be suspected in patients who have suffered a traumatic injury, or who have been in a violent accident (fall, automobile accident).
   - ☐ a. Broken leg.
   - ☐ b. Heart attack.
   - ☐ c. Cardiac arrest.
   - ☐ d. Head, neck, or back injury.

3. The modified jaw thrust lets the rescuer open the airway while keeping the patient's head _____.
   - ☐ a. Tilted backward.
   - ☐ b. Turned to the side.
   - ☐ c. From moving.
   - ☐ d. Tilted forward.

4. The following type of rescue breathing is used when the patient's jaw or mouth is injured:
   - ☐ a. Mouth-to-stoma.
   - ☐ b. Mouth-to-nose.
   - ☐ c. Mouth-to-mouth.
   - ☐ d. Mouth-to-ear.

Fill in the blank with the correct word(s).

5. Persons with a stoma breathe air directly into the _____, bypassing both the mouth and nose.

6. While giving rescue breathing, if the rescuer notices that the patient's stomach is distended, he or she should take the following steps:

a. Make sure the patient's head is _____ far enough.

b. Breathe into the patient only enough to make the _____ rise.

c. _____ between breaths long enough to let the patient's lungs empty and to take another breath.

7. When positioning the patient with a head, neck, or back injury, the head, neck, and back should be supported and turned as a _____.

Answers

1. **b.** A rescuer should use the **modified jaw thrust** to open the airway if he or she suspects that the patient has a head, neck, or back injury.

2. **d.** A **head, neck, or back injury** should always be suspected in patients who have suffered a traumatic injury, or who have been in a violent accident.

3. **c.** The modified jaw thrust lets the rescuer open the airway while keeping the patient's head **from moving.**

4. **b. Mouth-to-nose breathing** is used when the patient's jaw or mouth is injured.

5. Persons with a stoma breathe air directly into the **windpipe,** bypassing both the mouth and nose.

6. If a patient's stomach becomes distended during rescue breathing, the rescuer should:
   a. Make sure the patient's head is **tilted back** far enough.
   b. Breathe into the patient only enough to make the **chest** rise.
   c. **Pause** between breaths long enough to let the patient's lungs empty and to take another breath.

7. When positioning the patient with a head, neck, or back injury, the head, neck, and back should be supported and turned as a **unit.**

Practice Session: Rescue Breathing Using the Modified Jaw Thrust

Skill Sheet:

Survey the Scene

Look for mechanism of injury that might indicate a head, neck, or back injury.

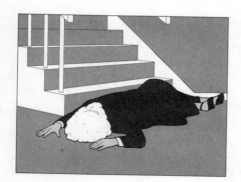

Stabilize the Patient's Head and Neck

Kneel behind the patient. Stabilize the patient's head (keep the head still) by placing your hands along both sides of the patient's head with the fingers touching the jaw line, to prevent the head from moving from side to side or forward and backward.

Check for Unresponsiveness

Ask (*do not shout*), "Are you OK?"

Call for Help

Position the Patient (It is recommended that more than one person help turn the patient.)

Caution must be observed in moving patients with suspected head, neck, or back injuries. Roll the patient so that the head, neck, and body move as one unit:

Kneel at patient's shoulders.

Straighten patient's legs, if necessary, and move patient's arm closest to you above patient's head.

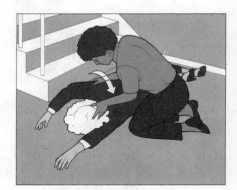

Place your hand closest to patient's head behind patient's head and neck for support.

With your other hand, grasp the patient under the other arm to keep the upper body aligned with the head and neck.

Using the hand under the arm, pull steadily and gently to roll the patient, while controlling the movement of the head and neck with the other hand as you turn the body as a unit.

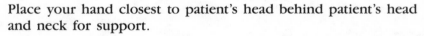

Open the Airway

Kneel at an angle behind the patient's head.

Rest your elbows on the surface on which the patient is lying.

Position your hands on both sides of the patient's head to keep it from moving from side to side or forward and backward.

Place the fingers of both hands along the patient's jawbone between the earlobes and angles of the jaw.

Position the thumbs across the patient's cheekbones.

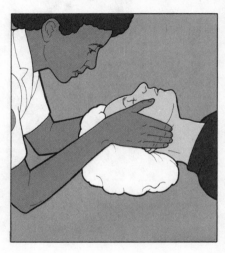

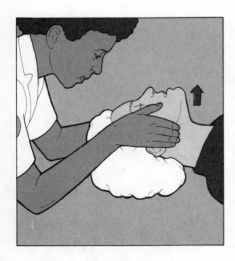

Apply pressure with fingers to the angles of the lower jaw to lift upward while maintaining pressure on the cheekbones.

At the same time, keep the head from moving backward with the palms of the hands.

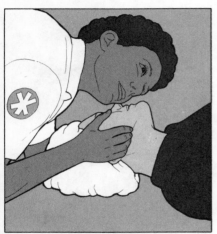

Check for Breathlessness

Maintain open airway using modified jaw thrust.

Look, listen, and feel for breathing for 3 to 5 seconds.

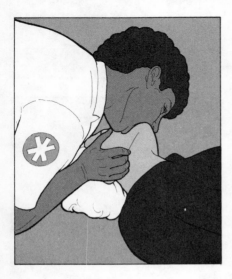

Give 2 Full Breaths

Maintain open airway using modified jaw thrust.

Close off patient's nostrils by pushing your cheek against patient's nose.

Make a tight seal around patient's mouth and give 2 full breaths at the rate of 1 to 1½ seconds per breath.

Observe chest rise and fall; listen and feel for escaping air.

Check for Pulse

Maintain in-line stabilization with one hand.

Locate Adam's apple with middle and index fingers of other hand.

Slide fingers from Adam's apple down into the groove of neck on the side closest to you.

Feel for carotid pulse for 5 to 10 seconds.

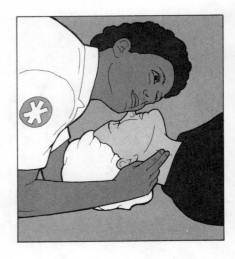

Phone the EMS System for Help

Tell someone to call an ambulance.

Rescuer says, "No breathing, has pulse, call _____" (local emergency number or Operator).

Begin Rescue Breathing

Give 1 breath every 5 seconds at the rate of 1 to 1½ seconds per breath.

Practice Session: Mouth-to-Nose Breathing

Skill Sheet:

Check for Unresponsiveness

Shout for Help

Position the Patient

Open the Airway

Check for Breathlessness

Give 2 Full Breaths:

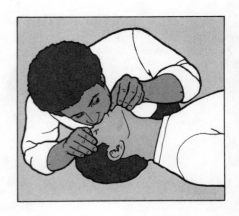

Maintain backward head-tilt position with one hand on the patient's forehead.

Use the other hand to close the patient's mouth, making sure to push on the chin and not on the throat.

Open your mouth wide, take a deep breath, and seal your mouth tightly around the patient's nose.

Give 2 full breaths at the rate of 1 to 1½ seconds per breath.

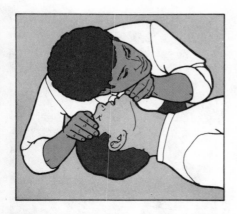

Open the patient's mouth between breaths in order to allow air to come out.

Observe chest rise and fall; listen and feel for escaping air.

Check for Pulse

Phone the EMS System for Help

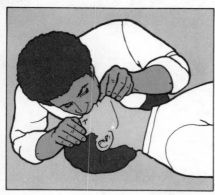

Begin Mouth-to-Nose Rescue Breathing

Maintain backward head-tilt position with one hand on the forehead.

Use the other hand to close the patient's mouth, making sure to push on the chin and not on the throat.

Open your mouth wide, take a deep breath, and seal your mouth tightly around the patient's nose.

Give 1 breath every 5 seconds at the rate of 1 to 1½ seconds per breath.

Open the patient's mouth between breaths in order to allow air to come out.

Observe chest rise and fall; listen and feel for escaping air.

Continue for 1 minute.

Recheck Pulse

Continue Rescue Breathing

Skill Checklist: Rescue Breathing Using the Modified Jaw Thrust

Critical Skill	Steps	PC	IC
Survey the Scene	Look for mechanism of injury that might indicate a head, neck, or back injury.		
Stabilize the Patient's Head	Kneel behind the patient. Stabilize the patient's head (keep the head still) by placing your hands along both sides of the patient's head with the fingers touching the jaw line, to prevent the head from moving from side to side or forward and backward.		
Check for Unresponsiveness	Ask, "Are you OK?"		
Call for Help	Call for help to attract another person's attention.		
Position the Patient (Use more than 1 rescuer)	Roll patient onto back if necessary: use caution when moving patients with suspected head, neck, or back injuries. Roll patient toward you as a unit; as you roll patient, support back of head and neck, and keep the upper body aligned with the head and neck.		
Open the Airway	Kneel at an angle behind the patient's head. Rest your elbows on the surface on which the patient is lying. Position your hands on both sides of the patient's head. Place the fingers of both hands along the patient's jawbone between the earlobes and angles of the jaw. Position the thumbs across the patient's cheekbones. Apply pressure with fingers to the angles of the lower jaw to lift upward while maintaining pressure on the cheekbones. Keep the head from moving backward.		
Check for Breathlessness	Maintain open airway using modified jaw thrust. Look at chest; listen and feel for breathing for 3 to 5 seconds.		
Give 2 Full Breaths	Maintain open airway using modified jaw thrust. Close off patient's nostrils by pushing your cheek against patient's nose. Give 2 full breaths.		
Check for Pulse	Maintain in-line stabilization with one hand. Feel for pulse for 5 to 10 seconds.		
Phone the EMS System for Help	Tell someone to call for an ambulance.		
Begin Rescue Breathing	Give 1 breath every 5 seconds.		
Decision Making	Based on the information the instructor gives, make a decision about what to do next, and continue giving the appropriate care.		

Final Instructor Check _____

Airway Management Skills Checklists

Skill Checklist: Mouth-to-Nose Rescue Breathing

Critical Skill	Steps	PC	IC
Begin Primary Survey	Check for unresponsiveness. Shout for help. Position the patient. Open the airway. Check for breathlessness.		
Give 2 Full Breaths	Maintain backward head-tilt with one hand on patient's forehead. Close patient's mouth. Seal your mouth around the patient's nose and give 2 full breaths. Open patient's mouth between breaths.		
Check for Pulse	Feel for carotid pulse for 5 to 10 seconds.		
Phone the EMS System for Help	Tell someone to call for an ambulance.		
Begin Mouth-to-Nose Rescue Breathing	Give mouth-to-nose rescue breathing. Give 1 breath every 5 seconds. Open patient's mouth between breaths.		
Recheck Pulse	Feel for carotid pulse for 5 seconds.		
Continue Mouth-to-Nose Rescue Breathing	Give 1 breath every 5 seconds.		
Decision Making	Based on the information the instructor gives, make a decision about what to do next, and continue giving the appropriate care.		

Final Instructor Check _____

8 Use of the Resuscitation Mask for Rescue Breathing

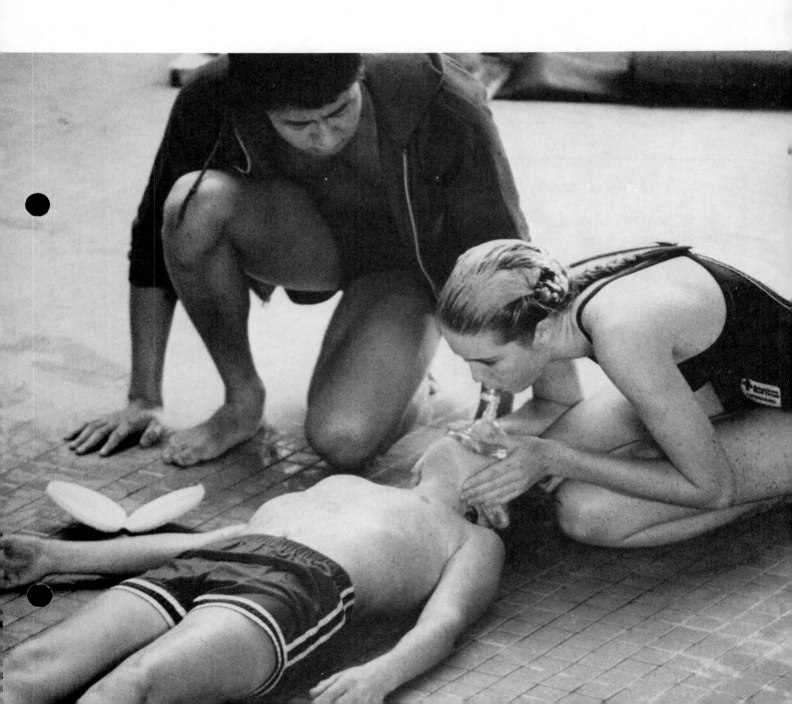

Use of the Resuscitation Mask for Rescue Breathing

MAIN IDEAS

1. The resuscitation mask is an effective aid for rescue breathing.
2. The resuscitation mask serves as a barrier between the rescuer and the patient.
3. The resuscitation mask has several advantages over other breathing equipment.
4. The resuscitation mask may be used for performing rescue breathing in one- or two-rescuer CPR.

CHAPTER OUTLINE

I. Purpose of the Resuscitation Mask
II. Advantages of the Resuscitation Mask
III. Using the Resuscitation Mask
   A. If the patient vomits
   B. Cleaning the mask
IV. Review
V. Practice Sessions
   A. Rescue breathing: triple airway maneuver
   B. Rescue breathing: modified jaw thrust
   C. Two-rescuer CPR

OBJECTIVES

1. Identify three advantages of using the resuscitation mask for rescue breathing.
2. Describe and demonstrate the use of the resuscitation mask.

Purpose of the Resuscitation Mask

A **resuscitation mask** is a transparent, semisoft, dome-shaped device that fits over the patient's mouth and nose, providing an aid to ventilation. It permits the rescuer to provide rescue breathing without mouth-to-mouth contact. Some masks, such as the Laerdal Pocket Mask™, are equipped with a one-way valve that permits air to enter the patient's airway and diverts exhaled air away from the rescuer.

For individuals who perform CPR frequently, there is a potential risk of disease transmission. The professional rescuer is taught to use the resuscitation mask because he or she may have to perform CPR frequently. There could be vomit, blood, or other body fluids around a victim's mouth due to regurgitation and/or trauma. The use of the resuscitation mask places a barrier between rescuer and patient by eliminating mouth-to-mouth and other facial contact.

Advantages of the Resuscitation Mask

The resuscitation mask permits the rescuer to deliver mouth-to-mask ventilation for adults, and, with certain masks, children and infants. In addition to providing a barrier, the mask, if used correctly:

- Permits air to travel through the patient's mouth and nose at the same time.

- Provides an adequate seal even in cases where the patient has serious facial injuries.

- Provides an alternative as effective or more effective than other methods of ventilation (for example, mouth-to-mouth and bag mask ventilation). Research has shown that the rescuer using a resuscitation mask can deliver a volume of air far beyond the minimum amount (800 ml) required for normal rescue breathing.

- Permits the rescuer to provide oxygen-enriched air to unconscious patients who are not breathing, and to conscious patients who require oxygen. (This can only be done with masks that have an oxygen inlet.)

Using the Resuscitation Mask

When using a resuscitation mask, such as the Laerdal Pocket Mask™, the rescuer takes the following steps:

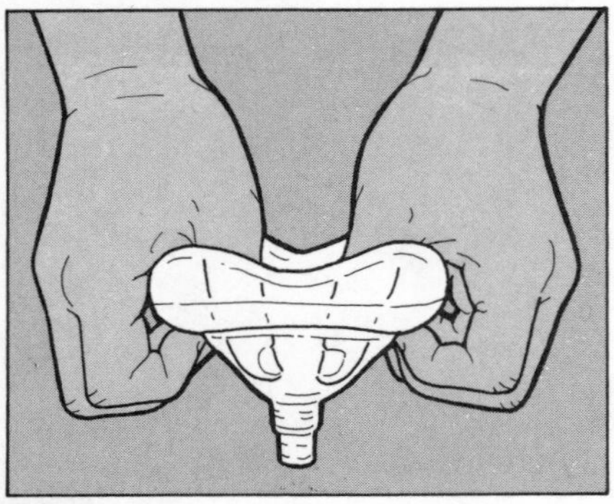

1. Opens the mask by pushing out the dome with the thumbs and forefingers of both hands *(Fig. 26)*.

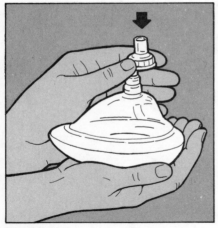

Figure 26
Pushing Out the Dome of the Mask

2. Places the one-way valve on the opening of the mask *(Fig. 27)*.

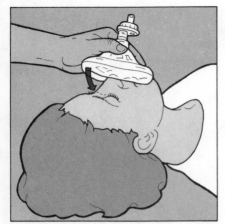

Figure 27
Placing the One-Way Valve on the Mask

3. Kneels behind the patient's head.

4. Places the mask on the patient by putting the rim of the mask between the patient's lower lip and chin *(Fig. 28)*.

Figure 28
Placing the Mask on the Patient

5. Brings the mask forward and applies pressure on it with the thumbs on each side of the mask so that the lower lip is pushed forward and the mouth is kept open under the mask.

6. Places the fingers of both hands along the patient's jawbone between the earlobes and the angles of the jaw *(Fig. 29)*.

7. Rests his or her elbows on the surface on which the patient is lying.

Note: For patients with possible head, neck, or back injuries, the modifed jaw thrust should be used to open the airway.

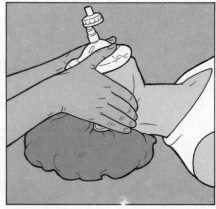
Figure 29
Placing the Fingers Along the Patient's Jawbone

8. Using the triple airway maneuver, lifts upward with the fingers while applying downward and forward pressure on the mask with thumbs and tilts the head back *(Fig. 30)*.

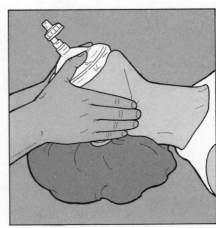
Figure 30
Triple Airway Maneuver With a Resuscitation Mask

9. Makes sure that the patient's mouth is open, and blows into the mask until the patient's chest rises *(Fig. 31)*.

10. Continues to maintain an open airway, watches the chest rise and fall, and breathes at the appropriate rate for adults, children, or infants.

Note: Directions for use of resuscitation masks vary from manufacturer to manufacturer. Some masks are not appropriate for use on children or infants. Be sure to consult manufacturer's directions for correct use.

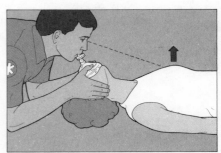
Figure 31
Breathing Into the Mask and Watching the Chest Rise

If the Patient Vomits

If the patient vomits while the resuscitation mask is in place, the rescuer removes the mask, turns the patient's head and body to the side as a unit, and uses finger sweeps to remove the vomit from the patient's mouth. If it can be done quickly, the rescuer empties the vomit from the mask, making sure the one-way valve is not clogged. Then the rescuer reapplies the mask to the patient's face and continues rescue breathing. The rescuer's first priority must be to continue to ventilate the patient in a timely manner, using mouth-to-mouth breathing or another mask if available.

Cleaning the Resuscitation Mask After Use

Manufacturer's instructions for cleaning the resuscitation mask should be followed after each use.

Usually, the disposable one-way valve on the resuscitation mask can be cleaned and reused after practice on a manikin. For use on a patient, the disposable one-way valve should not be reused. The resuscitation mask and one-way valve may be cleaned by first washing in warm soapy water and rinsing with clean water. Both are then submerged for 10 minutes in a solution of water and household bleach (2 ounces household bleach to 1 gallon of water). They are then rinsed with clean water and allowed to dry. The mask should not be pasteurized, boiled, or steamed (autoclaved).

Review

Check the correct answer.

1. The resuscitation mask permits air to travel—
   - ☐ a. Through the mouth only.
   - ☐ b. Through the mouth and nose.
   - ☐ c. Through the nose only.

2. The resuscitation mask—
   - ☐ a. Cannot be used for patients with facial injuries.
   - ☐ b. Provides an adequate seal for patients with facial injuries.

3. The resuscitation mask provides a barrier—
   - ☐ a. For the rescuer.
   - ☐ b. For the patient.
   - ☐ c. Between the rescuer and the patient.

4. When placing the mask on the patient, the rescuer—
   - ☐ a. Places the rim between the patient's lower lip and chin.
   - ☐ b. Places the rim over the chin in an adult.
   - ☐ c. Places the rim above the upper lip.

5. When the mask is in place and held with both thumbs, the rescuer places his or her fingers—
   - ☐ a. Over the patient's chin.
   - ☐ b. Under the patient's upper jaw.
   - ☐ c. Along the patient's jawbone between the earlobes and angles of the jaw.

6. The rescuer must be sure that—
   - ☐ a. The mouth is open under the mask at all times.
   - ☐ b. The airway is open.
   - ☐ c. The airway is open and the mouth is open under the mask.

Use of the Rescuscitation Mask for Rescue Breathing

Answers

1. **b.** The resuscitation mask permits air to travel **through the mouth and nose.**

2. **b.** The resuscitation mask **provides an adequate seal for patients with facial injuries.**

3. **c.** The resuscitation mask provides a barrier **between the rescuer and the patient.**

4. **a.** When placing the mask on the patient, the rescuer **places the rim between the patient's lower lip and chin.**

5. **c.** When the mask is in place and held with both thumbs, the rescuer places his or her fingers **along the patient's jawbone between the earlobes and angles of the jaw.**

6. **c.** The rescuer must be sure that **the airway is open and the mouth is open under the mask.**

Practice Session: Using the Resuscitation Mask for Rescue Breathing (Triple Airway Maneuver)

Skill Sheet:

Check for Unresponsiveness
Shout for Help

Position the Patient

Open the Airway
   Use the head-tilt/chin-lift method.

Check for Breathlessness

Position Mask for Rescue Breathing

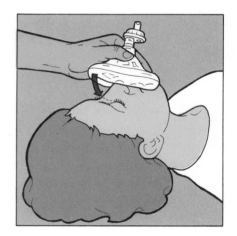

   If patient is not breathing, prepare resuscitation mask for use by pushing out the dome and attaching the one-way valve if provided.

   Kneel behind the patient's head.

   Place the rim of the mask between the patient's lower lip and chin.

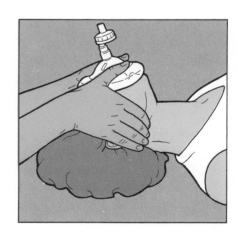

   Place your thumbs on each side of the mask so that the lower lip is pushed forward and the mouth is kept open under the mask.

   Place the fingers of both hands along the patient's jawbone between the earlobes and angles of the jaw.

   Rest your elbows on the surface on which the patient is lying.

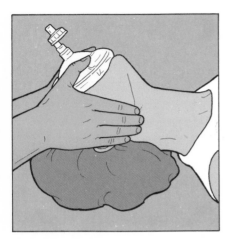

Lift upward with your fingers while you apply downward and forward pressure on the mask with your thumbs; tilt the head back (triple airway maneuver).

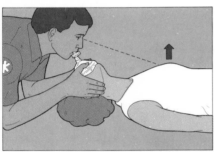

Give 2 Full Breaths

Take a deep breath and make a tight seal around the mouthpiece on the mask.

Give 2 full breaths at the rate of 1 to 1½ seconds per breath.

Observe chest rise and fall.

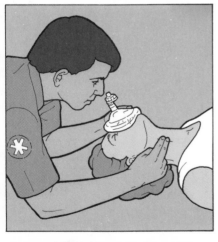

Check for Pulse

Maintain head-tilt with one hand on mask.

Locate Adam's apple with middle and index fingers of other hand.

Slide fingers down into groove of neck.

Feel for carotid pulse for 5 to 10 seconds.

Phone the EMS System for Help

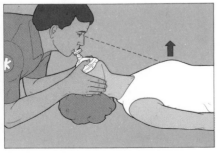

Begin Rescue Breathing

Give 1 breath every 5 seconds at the rate of 1 to 1½ seconds per breath.

Practice Session: Using the Resuscitation Mask for Rescue Breathing (Modified Jaw Thrust When Head, Neck, or Back Injury Is Suspected)

Skill Sheet:

Survey the Scene

Look for mechanism of injury that might indicate a head, neck, or back injury.

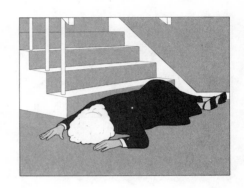

Stabilize the Patient's Head and Neck

Kneel behind the patient. Stabilize the patient's head (keep the head still) by placing your hands along both sides of the patient's head with the fingers touching the jaw line, to prevent the head from moving from side to side or forward and backward.

Check for Unresponsiveness

Ask (*do not shout*), "Are you OK?"

Call for help.

Position the Patient (It is recommended that more than one person help turn the patient.)

Caution must be observed in moving patients with suspected neck or back injuries. Roll the patient so that the head, neck, and body move as one unit.

Open the Airway

Use modified jaw thrust.

Check for Breathlessness

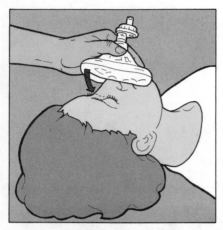

Position Mask for Rescue Breathing

If patient is not breathing, prepare resuscitation mask for use by pushing out the dome and attaching the one-way valve if provided.

Kneel behind the patient's head.

Place the rim of the mask between the patient's lower lip and chin.

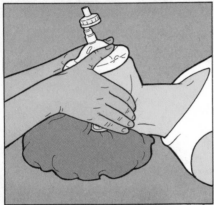

Place your thumbs on each side of the mask so that the lower lip is pushed forward and the mouth is kept open under the mask.

Place the fingers of both hands along the patient's jawbone between the earlobes and angles of the jaw.

Rest your elbows on the surface on which the patient is lying.

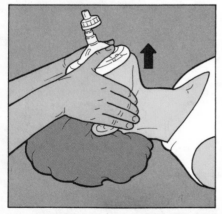

Lift upward with your fingers while you apply downward pressure on the mask with your thumbs (modified jaw thrust).

Note: The head should not be tilted back when a head, neck, or back injury is suspected. If the chest fails to rise during rescue breathing, the head should be tilted backward very slightly.

Give 2 Full Breaths

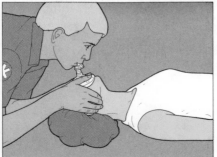

Take a deep breath and make a tight seal around the mouthpiece on the mask.

Give 2 full breaths at the rate of 1 to 1½ seconds per breath.

Observe the chest rise and fall.

Check for Pulse

Maintain in-line stabilization with one hand.

Locate Adam's apple with middle and index fingers of other hand.

Slide fingers down into groove of neck on side closest to you.

Feel for carotid pulse for 5 to 10 seconds.

Phone the EMS System for Help

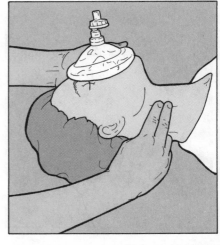

Begin Rescue Breathing

Give 1 breath every 5 seconds at the rate of 1 to 1½ seconds per breath.

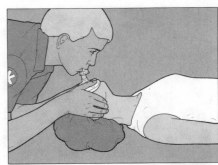

Practice Session: Two-rescuer CPR Using a Resuscitation Mask (Triple Airway Maneuver)

Skill Sheet:

First Rescuer (Ventilator)

Check for unresponsiveness.

Shout for help.

Position the patient.

Open the airway with head-tilt/chin-lift method.

Check for breathlessness.

Say, "No breathing."

Kneel behind patient's head.

Apply resuscitation mask using the triple airway maneuver.

Give 2 full breaths at the rate of 1 to 1½ seconds per breath.

Observe chest rise and fall.

Feel for carotid pulse for 5 to 10 seconds.

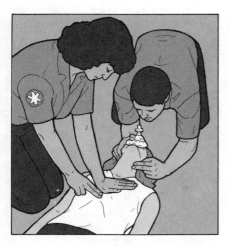

Second Rescuer (Compressor)

Kneel at patient's chest.

Locate landmark for chest compressions while first rescuer begins to check for pulse.

Assume correct hand position.

First Rescuer (Ventilator)

Say, "No pulse, begin CPR."

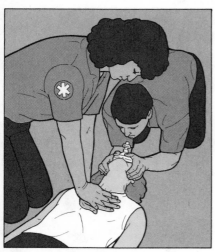

Second Rescuer (Compressor)

Begin chest compressions at a ratio of 5 compressions to 1 breath.

Stop after fifth compression to allow first rescuer to give 1 breath.

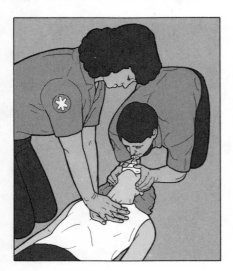

First Rescuer (Ventilator)

Give 1 full breath after every fifth compression.

Check compression effectiveness by checking pulse periodically while compressions are being given.

Say, "Pulse check" and feel for carotid pulse at end of first minute.

Recheck pulse every few minutes.

Skill Checklist: Using the Resuscitation Mask for Rescue Breathing (Triple Airway Maneuver)

Critical Skill	Steps	PC	IC
Begin Primary Survey	Check for unresponsiveness. Shout for help. Position the victim. Open the airway using the head-tilt/chin-lift method. Check for breathlessness.		
Position Mask for Rescue Breathing	Prepare resuscitation mask for use. Kneel behind the patient's head. Place the rim of the mask between the patient's lower lip and chin. Place your thumbs on each side of the mask so that the lower lip is pushed forward and the mouth is kept open under the mask. Place the fingers of both hands along the patient's jawbone between the earlobes and angles of the jaw. Rest your elbows on the surface on which the patient is lying. Lift upward with your fingers while you apply downward and forward pressure on the mask with your thumbs. Tilt the head back (triple airway maneuver).		
Give 2 Full Breaths	Make a tight seal around mouthpiece on mask. Give 2 full breaths.		
Check for Pulse	Feel for pulse for 5 to 10 seconds.		
Phone the EMS System for Help	Tell someone to call for an ambulance.		
Begin Rescue Breathing	Give 1 breath every 5 seconds.		
Decision Making	Based on the information the instructor gives, make a decision about what to do next, and continue giving the appropriate care.		

Final Instructor Check _____

Use of the Rescuscitation Mask for Rescue Breathing Skills Checklists

Skill Checklist: Using the Resuscitation Mask for Rescue Breathing (Modified Jaw Thrust)

Critical Skill	Steps	PC	IC
Survey the Scene	Look for mechanism of injury that might indicate head, neck, or back injury.		
Stabilize Patient's Head	Kneel behind the patient. Stabilize the patient's head (keep the head still) by placing your hands along the patient's head to prevent the head from moving from side to side or forward and backward.		
Check for Unresponsiveness	Ask, "Are you OK?"		
Call for Help	Call for help to attract another person's attention.		
Position the Patient (Use more than 1 rescuer)	Roll patient onto back if necessary: use caution when moving patients with suspected head, neck, or back injuries. Roll patient toward you as a unit; as you roll patient support back of head and neck, and keep the upper body aligned with the head and neck.		
Open the Airway	Use modified jaw thrust.		
Check for Breathlessness	Maintain open airway using modified jaw thrust. Look at chest; listen and feel for breathing for 3 to 5 seconds.		
Position Mask for Rescue Breathing	Prepare resuscitation mask for use. Kneel behind the patient's head. Place the rim of the mask between the patient's lower lip and chin. Place your thumbs on each side of the mask so that the lower lip is pushed forward and the mouth is kept open under the mask. Place the fingers of both hands along the patient's jawbone between the earlobes and angles of the jaw. Rest your elbows on the surface on which the patient is lying. Apply upward pressure with your fingers to the back of the jaw. Lift upward with your fingers while you apply downward pressure on the mask with your thumbs (modified jaw thrust). *Note:* The head should not be tilted back when a neck or back injury is suspected. If the chest fails to rise during rescue breathing, the head should be tilted backward very slightly.		
Give 2 Full Breaths	Make a tight seal around mouthpiece on mask. Give 2 full breaths.		
Check for Pulse	Maintain in-line stabilization with one hand. Feel for pulse for 5 to 10 seconds.		
Phone the EMS System for Help	Tell someone to call for an ambulance.		
Begin Rescue Breathing	Give 1 breath every 5 seconds.		
Decision Making	Based on the information the instructor gives, make a decision about what to do next, and continue giving the appropriate care.		

Final Instructor Check _____

Skill Checklist: Two-rescuer CPR Using a Resuscitation Mask (Triple Airway Maneuver)

Critical Skill	Steps	PC	IC
First Rescuer (Ventilator) Do a Primary Survey	Check for unresponsiveness. Shout for help. Position the patient. Open the airway using head-tilt/chin-lift method. Check for breathlessness. Apply resuscitation mask using triple airway maneuver. Give 2 full breaths. Feel for carotid pulse for 5 to 10 seconds.		
Second Rescuer (Compressor) Locate Compression Position Give 5 Compressions	Locate landmark for chest compressions while ventilator checks for pulse. Assume correct hand position. After ventilator says, "No pulse, begin CPR," give 5 compressions. Stop after fifth compression and allow ventilator to give 1 breath.		
Ventilator Give 1 Full Breath	After fifth compression, give 1 full breath.		
Do Compression/ Breathing Cycles	Do 12 cycles of 5 compressions and 1 breath. Ventilator monitors effectiveness of compressions by checking pulse while partner is compressing.		
Ventilator Recheck Pulse	Feel for carotid pulse for 5 seconds.		
Decision Making	Based on the information the instructor gives, make a decision about what to do next, and continue giving the appropriate care.		

Final Instructor Check _____

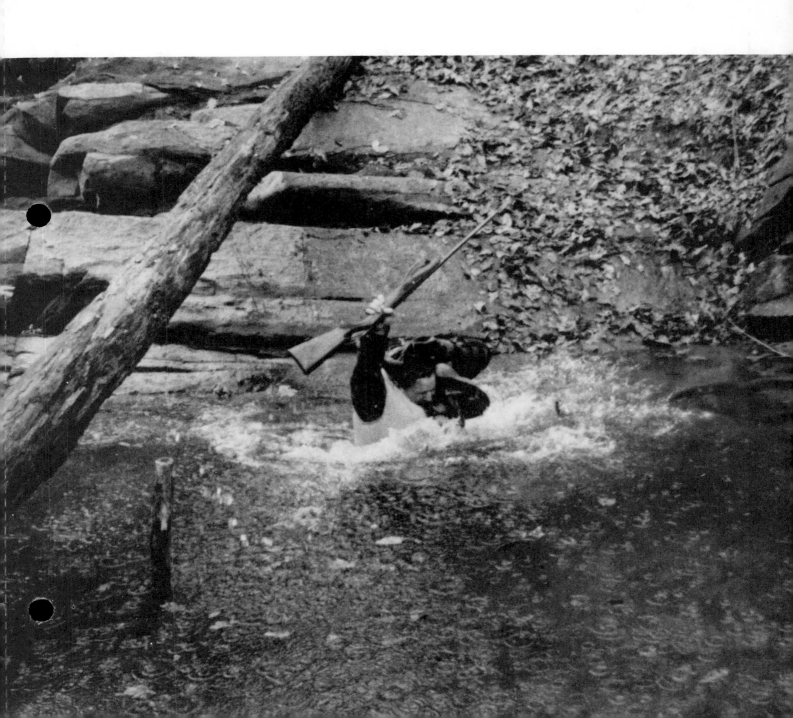

Special Resuscitation Situations

MAIN IDEAS

1. Certain situations require changes in the normal procedures used in providing basic life support (BLS).
2. These special situations include respiratory and/or cardiac arrest resulting from near drowning, traumatic injury, electric shock, and hypothermia.
3. Professional rescuers performing CPR are often required to work in unusual locations and situations that require modifications of normal BLS techniques.

CHAPTER OUTLINE

I. Providing Basic Life Support Under Special Conditions
II. Respiratory or Cardiac Arrest from—
   A. Near drowning
   B. Traumatic injury
   C. Electric shock
   D. Hypothermia (severe cold)
III. CPR in Difficult Locations and Situations
IV. Review

OBJECTIVES

1. Identify those special situations that require changes in normal BLS procedures.
2. Describe the special procedures used in giving BLS to victims of near drowning, traumatic injury, electric shock, and hypothermia.

Providing Basic Life Support Under Special Conditions

Sometimes there are situations that require the professional rescuer to modify emergency care procedures that are normally used in providing BLS. The four most common special situations are—
- Near drowning.
- Traumatic injury.
- Electric shock.
- Hypothermia (exposure to severe cold).

Each of these is discussed in this chapter, with information about modifications that need to be made when providing BLS. The chapter also describes giving CPR in difficult locations and situations.

Near Drowning

A person who has been submerged in water for more than 2 or 3 minutes will suffer from lack of oxygen and need emergency care. There are six steps in the management of a near-drowning victim.

Note: Rescuers attempting water rescue should be properly trained and wear a personal flotation device.

1. **Rescuing the Victim**
   The rescuer should get to the victim as quickly as possible without risking personal safety. If possible, the rescuer should use some sort of reaching or flotation device such as a pole, boat, surfboard, raft, life jacket, etc., to aid in the rescue.

2. **Rescue Breathing**
   Rescue breathing should be started as soon as possible, even before the patient is moved out of the water.

3. **Head, Neck, or Back Injuries**
   If there is any reason to suspect a head, neck, or back injury, such as a diving accident, the patient's head, neck, and back should be kept aligned. The patient should then be floated onto a backboard before being removed from the water. For example, a surfboard can be used for support and flotation.
   If a head, neck, or back injury is suspected, the rescuer uses the modified jaw thrust to open the airway. Rescue breathing should be given with the patient lying flat, without tilting his or her head backward, forward, or side to side.

4. **Clearing Water From the Airway**
   It is unnecessary to attempt to remove water from a patient's lungs or stomach. Only a small amount of water is aspirated by most drowning victims.

5. **Chest Compressions**
   Chest compressions should not be performed in the water, because the back needs firm horizontal support in order for

compressions to be effective. When the patient has been removed from the water, the rescuer should assess his or her breathing and circulation. The pulse may be difficult to detect in a victim of near drowning, and should be checked for up to 1 minute. If a pulse cannot be felt, CPR should be started at once.

6. **Additional Care**

   BLS should be continued until advanced cardiac life support (ACLS) personnel take over. Every near-drowning victim—even people who recover spontaneously or who require only minimal resuscitation—should be transported without delay to a medical facility for followup care.

   Even in cases where a victim of near drowning may have been in the water for a prolonged period, the rescuer should begin resuscitation. Patients have been successfully resuscitated after being submerged in cold water for longer than 30 minutes. CPR should be continued until advanced care can be started.

Traumatic Injury

According to the Standards and Guidelines, the survival rates from cardiac arrest due to trauma are generally poor. For this reason, the rescuer's emphasis should be on transporting such patients to a trauma center as soon as possible, so that specialized treatment can be directed to restoring blood flow and treating the traumatic injuries associated with the blood loss. Rescuers should pay special attention to the following:

1. **Not Moving the Patient**

   The professional rescuer should use care to avoid further injury to the patient at the scene of an accident. He or she should not try to remove an accident victim from an automobile unless there is immediate danger to the patient, such as from fire, flood, toxic fumes, etc., or unless the patient must be moved to provide CPR.

   Only those professional rescuers who have been trained in extrication procedures should attempt to remove the victim of an automobile accident who is pinned in a vehicle.

2. **Protecting the Head, Neck, and Back**

   The rescuer should suspect a head, neck, or back injury in trauma victims, particularly if the accident may have subjected his or her spine to sudden acceleration or deceleration (automobile accident, fall, diving, or skiing accident). The rescuer should do a primary survey, stabilize the patient's head, and do the modified jaw thrust to open the airway. (Procedures for conducting a primary survey on this type of patient are found in Chapter 7.)

3. Precautions for the Professional Rescuer

According to recent CDC guidelines, rescuers should avoid contact with blood and other body fluids when providing emergency care. Professional rescuers should read the guidelines for the prevention of disease transmission found at the beginning of Part II of this workbook on page 62, and consult with the course instructor for any changes.

Electric Shock

Electric shock can cause paralysis of the breathing muscles and cardiac arrest. It can also cause serious burns. The length of contact with electrical current, the strength of the current, and the environmental conditions are all factors related to the severity of injury. Rescuers should remember these rules:

1. Getting the Patient Clear

When attempting to rescue an electric shock victim, the rescuer must first make sure that such attempts will not endanger him or her, and then proceed to get the patient safely clear of the source of electricity. The person calling the EMS system should ask the dispatcher to call the power company if there are downed wires or power lines. Live wires should never be touched.

2. The ABCs

The patient's ABCs (**A**irway, **B**reathing, **C**irculation) must be checked at once, and rescue breathing or CPR must be started immediately if there is no breathing or pulse.

3. The Inaccessible Victim

A person who receives an electric shock when working in a high or hard-to-reach location, such as a public utility pole, should receive rescue breathing immediately, provided he or she is not in contact with the electrical source. The victim should be lowered to the ground if necessary, and CPR should be started as soon as possible. CPR is effective only when the patient is lying flat on a firm surface.

4. Lightning

Lightning acts as a direct current that interrupts the heart's rhythm. Victims most likely to die are those who suffer immediate cardiac arrest. Those whose hearts do not stop have the best chance of recovery. In addition, electric shocks often cause serious burns that require a physician's immediate attention. Advanced cardiac life support (ACLS) should follow basic life support for all electric shock victims.

Hypothermia (Exposure to Severe Cold)

Accidental **hypothermia** is a decrease in body temperature resulting from exposure to freezing or near-freezing temperatures. If the core temperature of the body falls below 95°F (35°C), symptoms of hypothermia will occur. Hypothermia decreases the flow of blood to the brain, lowers the body's oxygen requirements, causes blood pressure to fall, and can lead to cardiac arrest. The patient's pulse may be very difficult to feel, and he or she may appear to be dead.

Rescue breathing should be started right away if the patient is not breathing. Before starting CPR, the rescuer may need to check the patient's pulse for up to 1 minute. The patient should be transported immediately to a medical facility for followup care, with CPR continued on the way. Further heat loss from the body's core should be prevented by removing any wet clothing, rewarming the patient in warm dry clothing and blankets, and adding heat with hot water bottles and warm packs.

CPR in Difficult Locations and Situations

Whether they are performing two-rescuer or one-rescuer CPR, professional rescuers often find themselves working under unique or unusual circumstances. Professional rescuers have been known to perform CPR in bathrooms, in elevators, on subway platforms, and on moving buses. According to the Standards and Guidelines, situations that may occur and guidelines for how to handle them include:

1. **Changing Locations.** Patients are not moved from a cramped or busy location for convenience. They should only be moved if there is danger to rescuer or patient, or if it is impossible to perform CPR without moving the patient.

2. **Stairways.** In some instances a patient may have to be transported up or down a flight of stairs. It is best to perform CPR effectively at the head or the foot of the stairs and, at a predetermined signal, to interrupt CPR to move as quickly as possible to the next level, where CPR should be resumed. Interruptions should not last longer than 30 seconds and should be avoided if possible.

3. **Litters.** While transferring a patient into an ambulance or other mobile emergency care unit, CPR should not be interrupted—even when the person is actually being moved into the vehicle. The rescuer's need to give effective compressions and breaths should determine how quickly the litter is moved. With a low-wheeled litter, the rescuer can stand alongside, maintaining the locked-arm position for compression. With a high litter or bed, the rescuer may have to kneel beside the patient on the bed or litter to gain the height needed to compress the chest. If the patient is on a bed, a board will have to be positioned beneath the back to provide a firm surface against the mattress.

Review

Complete each of the following statements.

Near Drowning

1. Get to the victim as quickly as possible without risking personal _____.

2. Start rescue breathing as soon as possible before moving the patient out of the _____.

3. If a neck injury is suspected, keep the patient's head, neck, and back aligned and float him or her onto a

    _____.

4. Chest compressions should not be performed in the

    _____.

5. Every near-drowning patient should be transported without delay to a medical facility for followup _____.

Traumatic Injury

1. Unless there is immediate danger, only professional rescuers who have been trained in extrication procedures should _____ the victim of an automobile accident who is pinned in the vehicle.

2. A patient in cardiac arrest due to a traumatic injury should be transported to a _____ as soon as possible.

3. The _____ is used to open the airway if a head, neck, or back injury is suspected.

Special Resuscitation Situations

Electric Shock

1. The rescuer must be sure that rescue attempts will not endanger his or her own _____.

2. The rescuer must get the patient safely clear of the source of
_____.

3. A person who receives an electric shock in a high or hard-to-reach location should be lowered to the ground before
_____ is started.

Severe Cold (Hypothermia)

1. The patient's pulse may be difficult to _____.

2. Further heat loss is prevented by wrapping the patient in warm clothing and blankets, and adding
_____.

Difficult Locations and Situations

1. A patient found in a cramped space should not be moved unless there is not enough room to start _____.

2. CPR is _____ when a patient is being moved on a litter.

3. CPR is interrupted for no longer than _____ seconds when moving a patient up or down a stairway.

Answers

Near Drowning

1. Get to the victim as quickly as possible without risking personal **safety.**

2. Start rescue breathing as soon as possible before moving the patient out of the **water.**

3. If a neck injury is suspected, keep the patient's head, neck, and back aligned and float him or her onto a **backboard.**

4. Chest compressions should not be performed in the **water.**

5. Every near-drowning patient should be transported without delay to a medical facility for followup **care.**

Traumatic Injury

1. Unless there is immediate danger, only professional rescuers who have been trained in extrication procedures should **remove** the victim of an automobile accident who is pinned in the vehicle.

2. A patient in cardiac arrest due to a traumatic injury should be transported to a **trauma center** as soon as possible.

3. The **modified jaw thrust** is used to open the airway if a head, neck, or back injury is suspected.

Electric Shock

1. The rescuer must be sure that rescue attempts will not endanger his or her own **safety.**

2. The rescuer must get the patient safely clear of the source of **electricity.**

3. A person who receives an electric shock in a high or hard-to-reach location should be lowered to the ground before **CPR** is started.

Severe Cold (Hypothermia)

1. The patient's pulse may be difficult to **feel.**

2. Further heat loss is prevented by wrapping the patient in warm clothing and blankets, and adding **heat.**

Difficult Locations and Situations

1. A patient in a cramped space should not be moved unless there is not enough room to start **CPR.**

2. CPR is **continued** when a patient is being moved on a litter.

3. CPR is interrupted for no longer than **30** seconds when moving a patient up or down a stairway.

Footnotes

1. National Center for Health Statistics: Advance report of final mortality statistics, 1985. *Monthly Vital Statistics Report.* Vol. 36, No. 5, Supp. DHHS Pub. No. (PHS) 87–1120. Public Health Service. Hyattsville, Md., August 28, 1987.

2. Atkins, James M. 1986. Emergency Medical Service Systems in Acute Cardiac Care: State of the Art, *Circulation* 74 (Suppl. IV), IV–5.

3. Grant, Harvey D., Robert H. Murray, Jr., and J. David Bergeron, Fourth edition. 1986. *Emergency Care,* Englewood Cliffs, N.J.: Prentice-Hall, Inc.

4. *The Health Consequences of Smoking: Cardiovascular Disease: A Report of the Surgeon General.* 1983. Department of Health and Human Services publication 84-50204. U.S. Government Printing Office.

5. The Lipid Research Clinics Coronary Primary Prevention Trial Results: II. The Relationship of Reduction in Incidence of Coronary Heart Disease to Cholesterol Lowering. 1984. *JAMA,* 251:365–374.

Appendix

Medicolegal Considerations and Recommendations

Note: The American Red Cross advises professional rescuers to check with their employers and/or professional organizations to determine if there are specific state or local laws or standards of professional conduct that apply to them.

> The following guidelines have been excerpted with permission from the "Standards and Guidelines for Cardiopulmonary Resuscitation and Emergency Cardiac Care," reprinted from *The Journal of the American Medical Association,* June 6, 1986, Vol. 255, No. 21, pages 2979–2984. Copyright 1986, American Medical Association.

"The goal of the 1985 Conference participants was to ensure that these standards and guidelines for cardiopulmonary resuscitation (CPR) are the best possible based on scientific knowledge and medical practice. Legal liability may be based on either the quality of the care provided or the decision to provide, withhold, or withdraw care.[1] Providing high-quality care while maintaining sensitivity to the emotional needs and realities of patients and those close to them is the best way for care providers to avoid legal action . . .

Obligation to Provide CPR

"When a physician-patient relationship exists, the physician has an obligation to initiate CPR when medically indicated and when DNR status is not in force. Similarly, when nurses or paramedical persons are functioning in their official capacities, they have a positive obligation to initiate CPR when it is indicated. (In most states, the nurse and paramedic have been included in immunity statutes intended to protect them from liability for performing CPR out of the professional setting.)

"Thus, the accepted context in which a decision to withhold CPR may be made requires first that resuscitation can and will be implemented by a responsible person or agency if two conditions are fulfilled: (1) if there is the possibility that the brain is viable, and (2) if there is no legal or medical reason to withhold it. The first condition is determined by defining the presence or absence of brain death. The second provides for the possibility that resuscitation might not be indicated if it could do no good or if a competent refusal of CPR has been made . . .

Withdrawing BLS

"Nonphysicians should initiate CPR to the best of their knowledge and capability in cases they recognize as cardiac arrest. Nonphysicians who initiate BLS or advanced cardiac life support (ACLS) should continue resuscitation efforts until one of the following occurs: (1) effective spontaneous circulation and ventilation have been restored; (2) resuscitation efforts have been transferred to another responsible person who continues BLS; (3) a physician or a physician-directed person or team assumes responsibility; (4) the victim is transferred to properly trained personnel charged with responsibilities for emergency medical services; or (5) the rescuer is exhausted and unable to continue resuscitation . . .

Liability Risks of Individuals, Groups and Institutions

Immunity: 'Good Samaritan' Laws

"Good Samaritan laws have been expanded in a number of jurisdictions to protect almost every professional and layperson while that individual is acting 'in good faith' and is not guilty of gross negligence. An important purpose of such laws is to minimize fear of legal consequences for providing CPR and to eliminate this prohibitive fear in implementing a multilevel community ECC program.

Layperson Liability for CPR

"**Individual Rescuers.**—There has been no instance known to the 1985 Conference faculty and participants in which a layperson who has performed CPR reasonably has been sued successfully. There are a number of reasons why such a legal action is extremely unlikely in the future. These include (1) the provision of statutory immunity to laypersons as well as medical professionals in many jurisdictions for performance of CPR, in the form of Good Samaritan laws, and (2) the fact that successful prosecution of a layperson performing CPR in good faith would discourage, if not terminate, future layperson CPR and thus run counter to established public policy and interest. Laypersons are protected under most Good Samaritan laws if they perform CPR, even if they have had no formal training.

"Layperson CPR is beneficial for the cardiac arrest victim when performed in accordance with recognized standards. The BLS standards herein have been altered modestly to simplify teaching and remembering, thereby enhancing the confidence of the rescuer and, thus, the effectiveness of CPR.

"All citizens reasonably able to perform CPR, and for whom such performance does not pose a medical or psychoemotional danger, should be trained in and capable of performing CPR at a level to sustain the life of the cardiac and/or respiratory arrest victim until definitive therapy becomes available.

"**CPR Teachers and Organizations.**—People who are trainers in CPR are also protected under many Good Samaritan laws, as are organizations that sponsor this training, i.e., the American Heart Association (AHA), the American Red Cross, and similar agencies. The concern for liability for layperson CPR should not represent an impediment to full implementation of ECC capability . . .

Medicolegal Considerations in the Pediatric Age Group
(Decision-Making for Infants and Children)

Conclusions

"The student of BLS and ACLS must know the following about the ethical and legal obligations, particularly with respect to pediatric subjects, that attend lifesaving skills . . .:

- Where there exists substantial doubt about the authority or reasonableness of guardian requests to withhold CPR, a prescription in favor of resuscitation should govern professional conduct until a resolution of conflict can be achieved.
- Similarly, where potential rescuers are unsure of their pediatric skills, they should nevertheless undertake good faith efforts at resuscitation to the limit of their ability, relying on legal protection based on common law doctrines or Good Samaritan statutes. . . ."

Footnote

[1] McIntyre, K.M. Medicolegal aspects of decision-making in resuscitation and life support. Cardiovasc Rev. Rep. 1983; 4:46–56.

Glossary

Advanced Cardiac Life Support (ACLS): Use of special medical procedures and equipment to establish and/or maintain effective respiration and circulation for the victim of a cardiac emergency. Part of emergency cardiac care (ECC). *(Chapter 1)*

Airway: The passageway through which air enters the body and goes to the lungs. *(Chapter 3)*

Alveoli: Tiny air sacs in the lungs where oxygen and carbon dioxide are exchanged. *(Chapter 3)*

Aneurysm: A weak spot in an artery wall that bulges under pressure. *(Chapter 4)*

Angina Pectoris: Pain in the chest caused by insufficient oxygen to the heart, usually occurring during exercise, exertion, or stress. When blood vessels are narrowed due to atherosclerosis, and exertion causes the heart to require more oxygen, blood flow to the heart is restricted, causing pain. The pain of angina usually lasts only 2 to 10 minutes, unlike the pain of heart attack. *(Chapter 4)*

Arteries: Vessels that carry oxygen-rich blood away from the heart to the cells of the body. *(Chapter 3)*

Aspirate: Inhale foreign material into the lungs. *(Chapter 7)*

Atherosclerosis: A buildup of fatty substances such as cholesterol on the walls of the arteries, which causes the arteries to thicken and harden. *(Chapter 4)*

Basic Life Support (BLS): The level of care necessary to maintain a patient's breathing and circulation during a life-threatening emergency. BLS includes rescue breathing, CPR, the obstructed airway maneuver, and, where necessary, contacting the emergency medical services (EMS) system. (It also can include controlling bleeding and other lifesaving techniques.) *(Chapter 1)*

Bronchi: Branches of the windpipe that lead into the lungs. *(Chapter 3)*

Bystander CPR: See "Citizen CPR." *(Chapter 2)*

Capillaries: Small vessels where oxygen is transferred to tissues and exchanged for waste products such as carbon dioxide. *(Chapter 3)*

Cardiac Arrest: The condition in which the heart stops beating. *(Chapters 1 and 4)*

Cardiac Emergency: A life-threatening condition in which the heart is not functioning properly, such as a heart attack or cardiac arrest. *(Chapter 1)*

Cardiopulmonary Resuscitation (CPR): An emergency procedure used for a person who is not breathing and whose heart has stopped beating. The procedure involves a combination of rescue breathing and chest compressions. *(Chapters 1 and 3)*

Cardiovascular Disease: Any disease of the heart or blood vessels. *(Chapters 1 and 4)*

Cerebral Embolism: A blood clot that travels through the bloodstream and eventually blocks an artery in the brain. *(Chapter 4)*

Cerebral Thrombosis: A blood clot that forms in an artery in the brain and eventually blocks blood flow in the brain. *(Chapter 4)*

Cerebral Vascular Accident (CVA): Another term for stroke. *(Chapter 4)*

Cholesterol: A substance that causes a buildup of fatty deposits on the walls of arteries. Cholesterol is found in certain foods and is also produced by the body. *(Chapter 4)*

Citizen CPR: CPR delivered in an emergency by a citizen or layperson who has been trained to deliver basic CPR. Also called "bystander CPR" and "layperson CPR." *(Chapter 2)*

Coronary Heart Disease: A type of cardiovascular disease that affects the blood vessels of the heart. Blockages occurring in the blood vessels of the heart can lead to heart attack or cardiac arrest. *(Chapter 1)*

Glossary

Critical Skills: For the purposes of this course, the skills that participants must demonstrate correctly in order to pass the skill tests. Critical skills appear in the skill checklists. *(Chapters 5–8)*

Defibrillation: Application of an external electric shock to the heart to re-establish its regular electrical activity and restore an effective heartbeat. *(Chapters 1 and 4)*

Embolism: The condition in which a clot travels to an artery and blocks it. *(Chapter 4)*

Emergency Cardiac Care (ECC): All care that deals with cardiac emergencies. ECC includes recognizing the early warning signs of heart attack, providing BLS and ACLS as quickly as possible, and transporting the patient to a hospital for continued care. *(Chapter 2)*

EMS Dispatcher: A member of the emergency medical services (EMS) system team who receives emergency calls and dispatches (orders) the appropriate personnel and equipment to the scene of a medical emergency. *(Chapter 2)*

Emergency Medical Services (EMS) System: A community-based system that delivers specialized care to patients who are ill or injured. Care is provided at the scene of the emergency and is continued during transportation and following arrival at an appropriately staffed and equipped health care facility. *(Chapters 1 and 2)*

Epiglottis: A small valve over the trachea that helps keep out food and liquid. *(Chapter 3)*

Esophagus: The passageway that carries food and liquids to the stomach. *(Chapter 3)*

Exhalation: Expelling used air from the lungs through the airway. *(Chapter 3)*

Gastric Distention: Enlargement (distention) of the stomach caused by air entering the stomach, as may occur during rescue breathing. *(Chapter 7)*

Heart Attack: A condition in which blood flow to part of the heart is blocked, causing that part of the heart to die from lack of oxygen. *(Chapters 1 and 4)*

Hemorrhage: Sudden heavy bleeding. *(Chapter 4)*

High Blood Pressure: See "Hypertension."

Hypertension: A condition in which the pressure of blood flowing through the vessels of the circulatory system is higher than normal (also referred to as "high blood pressure"). *(Chapter 4)*

Hypothermia: Unintentional decrease in body temperature resulting from exposure to freezing or near-freezing temperatures. *(Chapter 9)*

Inhalation: Taking air into the lungs. *(Chapter 3)*

Larynx: Part of the upper trachea that contains the vocal cords. *(Chapter 3)*

Layperson CPR: See "Citizen CPR."

Modified Jaw Thrust: A method of opening the airway that minimizes movement of the neck and head. Used for patients with possible head, neck, or back injuries. *(Chapter 7)*

Myocardial Infarction (MI): Another term for heart attack. (Literally means "death of the heart muscle.") *(Chapter 4)*

Myocardium: The heart muscle. *(Chapter 4)*

Nitroglycerin: Frequently prescribed to relieve the pain of angina pectoris, this medication works to dilate (enlarge) the blood vessels so that blood flows more easily, and thus provides greater circulation of oxygen-carrying blood to the heart. *(Chapter 4)*

Pharynx: The common passageway for air and food leading from the back of the mouth, nose, and nasal passages to the trachea and esophagus. *(Chapter 3)*

Plaque: Accumulation of fatty deposits on artery walls that develops in atherosclerosis. *(Chapter 4)*

Professional Rescuer: A health or safety professional, working either in a volunteer or a paid position, who has a responsibility when on the job to assist an ill or injured person in a medical emergency. *(Chapter 1)*

Regurgitation: Vomiting. *(Chapters 7 and 8)*

Rescue Breathing: The process of breathing air into the lungs of a patient who has stopped breathing. *(Chapter 3)*

Respiratory Arrest: A condition in which breathing stops. *(Chapter 1)*

Respiratory Emergency: A condition in which normal breathing is difficult, or breathing stops. *(Chapter 1)*

Resuscitation Mask: A transparent, semisoft, dome-shaped device used to provide rescue breathing to a patient. The mask fits over the patient's mouth and nose. *(Chapter 8)*

Risk Factors: Conditions and behaviors that increase the likelihood of a person developing a disease. Some risk factors for cardiovascular disease cannot be changed. Others relate to lifestyle and can be changed. *(Chapter 4)*

Sternum: Breastbone. *(Chapter 3)*

Stroke: A condition in which one or more of the blood vessels in the brain becomes clogged or bursts, causing a part of the brain to die from lack of oxygen. *(Chapter 4)*

Thrombosis: The formation or presence of a clot within a blood vessel. *(Chapter 4)*

Trachea: The passageway that carries air from the larynx to the bronchi (also known as the windpipe). *(Chapter 3)*

Trauma: Physical injury usually caused by forceful impact. *(Chapters 7 and 9)*

Triple Airway Maneuver: A method of opening the airway in which the rescuer tilts the patient's head back, lifts the jaw upward, and opens the patient's mouth. The triple airway maneuver is also used when applying a resuscitation mask. *(Chapters 7 and 8)*

Veins: Vessels that carry de-oxygenated blood back to the heart and the lungs from the capillaries. *(Chapter 3)*

Ventricular Fibrillation: Chaotic, uncoordinated electrical activity of the heart that keeps it from pumping effectively. *(Chapter 4)*

Windpipe: See "Trachea."

Index

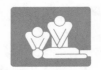

Index

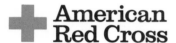 **American Red Cross**

Comparing BLS Skills

	ADULT (9 years and older)	CHILD (1–8 years)	INFANT (Under 1 year)
Rescue Breathing	• Give 1 breath every 5 seconds. • 1–1½ seconds per breath. • One minute = about 12 breaths.	• Give 1 breath every 4 seconds. • 1–1½ seconds per breath. • One minute = about 15 breaths.	• Give 1 breath every 3 seconds. • 1–1½ seconds per breath. • One minute = about 20 breaths.
Conscious Choking	• Determine if patient is choking. • Stand behind patient and deliver abdominal thrusts. • Repeat until object is expelled or patient loses consciousness.	• Determine if child is choking. • Stand or kneel behind child and deliver abdominal thrusts. • Repeat until object is expelled or child loses consciousness.	• Determine if infant is choking. • Give 4 back blows. • Give 4 chest thrusts. • Repeat until object is expelled or infant loses consciousness.
Unconscious Choking	• Give 2 full breaths. • Retilt head and give 2 full breaths. • Perform 6–10 abdominal thrusts. • Do finger sweep. • Give 2 full breaths. • Repeat abdominal thrusts, finger sweep, and 2 full breaths.	• Give 2 slow breaths. • Retilt head and give 2 slow breaths. • Perform 6–10 abdominal thrusts. • Do foreign body check. • Give 2 slow breaths. • Repeat abdominal thrusts, foreign body check, and 2 slow breaths.	• Give 2 slow breaths. • Retilt head and give 2 slow breaths. • Give 4 back blows. • Give 4 chest thrusts. • Do foreign body check. • Give 2 slow breaths. • Repeat back blows, chest thrusts, foreign body check, and 2 slow breaths.
One-rescuer CPR	• Depth of compression is 1½–2 inches. • Compressions are performed with both hands. • Compression rate: 80–100 per minute. • Do cycles of 15 compressions and 2 breaths.	• Depth of compression is 1–1½ inches. • Compressions are performed with one hand. • Compression rate: 80–100 per minute. • Do cycles of 5 compressions and 1 breath.	• Depth of compression is ½–1 inch. • Compressions are performed with two fingers. • Compression rate: 100–120 per minute. • Do cycles of 5 compressions and 1 breath.
Two-rescuer CPR	• Depth and rate of compressions are the same as one-rescuer CPR. • Do cycles of 5 compressions and 1 breath.	• Depth and rate of compressions are the same as one-rescuer child CPR. • Do cycles of 5 compressions and 1 breath.	• (Two-rescuer CPR is not used for infants.)

American Red Cross CPR: Basic Life Support for the Professional Rescuer